SO YOU WANT TO HAVE A BABY?

Tony Bradman

So you want to have a baby?

Julia MacRae

A DIVISION OF FRANKLIN WATTS

For Sally and our children

© 1985 Tony Bradman
All rights reserved
First published in Great Britain 1985 by
Julia MacRae Books. A division of Franklin Watts
12A Golden Square, London, W1R 4BA
and Franklin Watts Australia
1 Campbell Street
Artarmon, N.S.W.2064.

Typesetting by
The Word Factory, Rossendale, Lancashire
Printed in Great Britain by A. Wheaton & Co. Ltd, Exeter

British Library Cataloguing in Publication Data

Bradman, Tony
So you want to have a baby?
1. Pregnancy   2. Childbirth
I. Title
618.2   RG524

ISBN 0–86203–168–0 Hardback edition
ISBN 0–86203–212–1 Paperback edition

Contents

Acknowledgments vi

First words 7

1. Introduction 9

Part 1. **Before you have your baby** 15
2. Choices 17
3. Healthy parents, healthy babies 32

Part 2. **From conception to birth** 49
4. Conception 51
5. Being pregnant 68
6. Giving birth 90

Part 3. **Beginning to be a parent** 115
7. Home with your baby 117
8. How your child develops 139
9. Surviving parenthood 162

Last words 183
10. Is it worth it? 185

Further information 188

Index 189

Acknowledgments

THIS IS my first book, and I'd like to thank all the people who have helped me in writing it. Special thanks are due first of all to the three experts who have checked various parts of the manuscript for me: namely, Consultant Paediatrician, Dr Robert Dinwiddie, who checked Chapter 8; Consultant Obstetrician and Gynaecologist, Mr Cyril Young, who checked the other sections of the book which touch on medical matters; and Wendy Rose-Neil, my editor at *Parents*, who checked the sections dealing with nutrition. I would only add that all the opinions expressed are mine, as are any errors which may remain.

I would also like to express my deep gratitude to Julia MacRae for having the vision to commission a book like this, and also for having the patience to work with me on it through a difficult year. Special mention must also go to Richard and Angie Hill of the School Bookshop Association, and Pat Triggs, Editor of the SBA's magazine *Books for Keeps*, without whose help and encouragement this book wouldn't exist.

I'd also like to express my thanks to everyone connected with *Parents* now and in the past, and also to all the other people who are too numerous to mention but who have helped me greatly.

Most of all I'd like to thank my mother, my sister and her husband and children, and everyone else in my family for all their support and love.

First Words

1. Introduction

EVEN BEFORE my wife, Sally, and I got married, we had, like many other young couples, spent a lot of time talking about having children. Without thinking about it very clearly, we were both convinced that it was something we would inevitably do. Looking back, I'm sure we also thought simply feeling that way would get us off to a flying start as parents – when the day came.

Little did we know.

Three months after the wedding, we began to realise that our own personal transition to parenthood was on the way. If it sounds a little soon, it was – and it was unplanned. Or almost unplanned. It wasn't that we hadn't been using contraception; it was more that now we were married, it didn't seem important to use it carefully, especially as we intended to become parents eventually. We had therefore done what many other couples have done in the past – we had played 'fertility roulette' and won. Or had we lost?

It was when the pregnancy was confirmed that I think we both started to wonder what we'd let ourselves in for. Sally was immediately swept into a round of visits to the doctor and, later on, the hospital antenatal clinic. She had to cope with the common problems of early pregnancy, such as nausea and extreme tiredness. Soon, her body seemed to take on an independent life of its own as our baby grew within her and her front expanded. I, meanwhile, was trying to come to terms with the prospect of becoming a father – and being our family's sole breadwinner. It seemed an enormous change in our lives was about to happen in a very short space of time; one moment we were free and easy and the next we were to be Mum and Dad, with all the implications those names have.

That transition did happen very soon. Our beautiful baby daughter was born, and no one who is present at the birth of a child ever forgets it. Even though I'm going to try and describe the emotions of people who have been through it, in the end, those feelings are quite literally indescribable. The births of your children – especially your first child – are life-changing events, with a magic and a momentum all their own.

I will never forget the first few days after Sally came home from the hospital with our daughter, Emma. That's when it really hit both of us – and Emma too, probably – that we had done something we couldn't undo, and which was going to change our lives forever. We couldn't go back to the way things had been before; now there was a baby to be taken into account. It wasn't long before we realised that Emma's presence in our lives affected everything – and also that it was going to take us time to understand and cope with all the changes, if we ever managed it completely. In short, in those first few days of parenthood, we discovered what millions of parents have found out before – having a baby changes your life. It does so totally, and very, very suddenly.

On that very first day, everything went wrong, almost from the moment Sally came through the door holding our new baby. And when I say everything, I mean it. For instance, Emma started crying as soon as she came into our tiny flat, almost as if to say that she didn't think we could cope with looking after her on our own.

We also discovered that the plastic pants we had bought to put on over her nappies were too big for her – by a long way – so every time she unleashed her bladder she soaked everything in sight: her cot, its blankets and sheets, our bed and its bed clothes, the carpets, the furniture, me, Sally, everything. By two o'clock in the morning both Sally and I were beginning to think that perhaps having a baby wasn't such a good idea after all. And Emma was still crying.

I'm writing these words on the day of my daughter's fifth birthday. She's now a boisterous schoolgirl who can – and does – talk anybody to a standstill, including me, which is no mean feat. Sally and I survived, and Emma survived our incompetence. As parents, we learnt our trade with Emma, and even enjoyed the experience enough to go into it all over again with our second daughter, Helen; and go on to have a third child, our son Thomas.

1. Introduction

We survived; but things would have been a lot easier, and we would have got a lot more out of parenthood at that time, if we'd had some idea of what was coming *before* it happened. In those early months of Emma's life Sally and I kept saying to each other things like: "Why didn't anybody tell us that babies made so much washing? Why didn't anybody tell us that babies wake up in the middle of the night and won't go back to sleep, and that they can keep this sort of thing up for months on end? Why didn't anyone tell us just how much of a shock it would all be?"

Nobody told *me*, and that's for sure. I had had a few sex education classes at school, and I'd read some books on the subject. But they all stopped short at the point where the baby was conceived. They didn't tell me much at all about things like how a baby grows in the womb, how a woman's body changes during pregnancy, how birth happens or what it's like, or what effect having a baby has on your life. They certainly didn't tell me that having a baby would change my life as dramatically as it did.

Worst of all, I'd never read a book which tried to explain how I would *feel* about all this while it was happening; how I would worry, feel guilty, responsible, burdened, frightened, frustrated, bored at times – and at others ecstatic, tickled pink, happy, over the moon – and 1001 other things. I talked to people who'd been through it, too – my own parents, relatives, friends; but they weren't very much help either. It almost seemed as if there was a conspiracy of silence.

So I decided a long time ago that I would write the book we had needed and never had. I wanted it to be the book which would deal with all the questions which occur to you before you have a baby, questions like: "Is it worth it?" "How painful is birth, and will I ever be the same again?" "Isn't having a baby the complete end of your independence? No more freedom, no more social life, just boring old Mum and Dad?" I also wanted it to answer all the questions which start to crop up once you find yourself swept into the process of becoming a parent. I wanted it to help new parents to avoid some of that feeling of shock which hits you when you sit down at home with your own first baby and start to wonder what on earth you do next (see Chapter 7!).

And at last, I've managed to do it. I would have done it sooner, but I was too busy doing all the things parents have to do, like earning a living to support my family and enjoying the first years of my children's lives. For a large part of that time I've been working for a magazine called *Parents*, which is designed to do many of the things I'm aiming to do in this book. The difference is that here the advice and information is all under one roof, so to speak, while in a magazine it tends to be scattered over different issues.

At any rate, it's through my experiences working at *Parents* that I've come to realise there is a real need for a book like this. Many, many young parents go through the same problems that Sally and I did, and feel just as depressed, lonely and worried. More importantly, there are some young parents for whom the strain is too much, and who find themselves in very difficult circumstances. Severe depression, the breakdown of marriages, even family violence – such as baby battering – are far more common in families where the parents are younger than average and have little knowledge or experience of children. Much of the blame for problems like this must lie with the rosy, romantic illusions about parenthood fostered in our society. This book is designed to shatter those illusions and tell you what parenthood is really like.

It's for these reasons among others that I've put such a lot of thought and planning into the writing of this book. I want it to be useful to as many people as possible – those of you who are many years away from having children and may not even have decided whether you want to or not, as well as those who are either set on taking the first step towards parenthood, or who have already taken it.

What follows is divided into three sections. The first is called *Before you have your baby*, and looks at the reasons people put forward for wanting to have children. It also looks at how you can make sure you're both physically and emotionally *ready* to have a baby before you get pregnant, something which is very important indeed.

Part 2 is called *From conception to birth* and looks at the whole process of having a baby, from the moment when new life is created, to the day your baby is delivered. In this section you'll find out something else which very few sex education books even mention; that the growth and development of a baby in the womb is nothing short of miraculous, and fascinating in every detail. You'll also find out all about how both men and women react to pregnancy both physically and emotionally, and what birth is really like – in the words of people who have experienced it.

Part 3 is called *Beginning to be a parent*, and it's all about the practicalities of life with a young baby; the sleepless nights, the nappies, breastfeeding – and even the fun. It's also about how babies and children develop, and how you can make sure that your experience of parenthood is enjoyable, rewarding and satisfying for all of you – mother, father and children. I've also included some discussion of how society is slowly beginning to change in its attitudes towards women and families, and how this may affect your life.

So in what follows I hope you'll find all the information you'll need to understand parenthood and get the best out of it. I believe that it's the most rewarding thing many of us can do in our lives – and that you need to be prepared for it. I believe that having a baby is a great adventure, and the closest any of us ever comes to experiencing a real miracle. I think there's nothing like it in the world, and I wouldn't have missed it for anything. If you're like me, I hope this book will help you to decide for yourself whether you really want to have a baby – and then enjoy it if you do.

A note on sexes

You might think it odd that a book about having a baby should be written by a man. I've found out what I know about the subject through my work on *Parents* and simply through 'front-line' experience. I also believe that it's important for men to be as fully involved in the process of becoming a parent as women – and that in the future parenthood should be something shared between mothers *and* fathers. I'll be talking about that in greater detail further on. Suffice it to say here that this book is aimed equally at both halves of the human race – males and females.

One other thing which you might think a bit odd as you read on is that whenever I have to refer to a baby I use the words *she, her* and *hers*. That's partly because I'm used to thinking about babies as girls (the result of having two daughters). There's also a more conscious reason. In the many baby books I've read, babies are assumed more often than not to be male, and I think it's time girls got more of a look in. After all, it's the girls who actually have to go through the hardest part of having a baby! But most of what I say applies equally to boys and girls, and where it doesn't, I say so.

Part 1. **Before you have your Baby**

2. Choices

HAVING A BABY is the oldest, most basic fact of human existence. Everyone starts off in the same way, as a tiny scrap of living flesh in a woman's womb. That tiny scrap of flesh is a fertilised egg, the result of a fusion between a man's sperm and a woman's egg, two things which are brought together by sexual intercourse – the act of love.

The facts of life are that simple. They've always been that way, and even though scientists can produce 'test tube babies' and talk of all sorts of things like cloning and genetic engineering, they're still the same. Just as all the kings and queens and popes and presidents of history were created, just as Shakespeare, Karl Marx, Adolf Hitler, Albert Einstein, Mother Teresa and Joan of Arc were, so are human babies today.

But things have changed in a very fundamental way – and that only in recent years. Throughout most of mankind's history, men and women have had very little *choice* about whether or not to have children. Sex is a powerful, basic need, and it's powerful because it represents an instinctive, biological urge in us which we share with all living creatures; the urge to reproduce ourselves, to keep our particular species going.

What's different now is that we can interfere with that urge. We have methods of *contraception* which allow us to make love yet still make sure that it doesn't lead to having a baby. There's the pill, which is almost one hundred per cent effective in preventing pregnancy. There are the barrier methods, like the condom and Dutch cap. There are the intra-uterine devices like the coil which are also very effective. Even if your religion is opposed to these forms of contraception, there are the so-called natural methods, most of which involve working out when it's most 'dangerous' to have sex and avoiding intercourse on those days.

Before reliable methods of contraception were invented, couples had to face the possibility that each time they made love it could lead to pregnancy. So they were caught in a trap; most people needed sex, and sex almost always led to children, whether they were wanted or not.

Really effective contraception has only become a reality in this century – the pill, for example, only came into use in the United States in the 1950s, and in Britain in the early 1960s – and there are still many parts of the world where contraceptives aren't widely available. This is usually either because of economic problems or religious opposition, and for the people who live in those countries, there is still little choice about having children.

But contraception has made those of us who live in the rich, developed countries very fortunate people indeed. It means that we can choose *not* to have children if we don't want to. It means that we can choose how many children to have, and when to have them. It means that we can decide how big an age gap there should be between the children we have. All this gives us more freedom, and in particular one freedom that no other ages in human history have had; the freedom to make every child a *wanted* child.

It's probable that few children in the past were wanted in the way we can want a child now. Children just happened, like the weather; there was nothing you could do about it. Big families were common, as they still are in those parts of the world where contraception isn't easily available. Big families mean a strain on parents; on the mother, first and foremost, because her body is subjected to the physical stresses of endless pregnancy and childbirth, but on the father too, because he'll have to work to support an ever-growing number of hungry mouths. Big families and terrible poverty often go hand in hand. The children are affected, too; every child needs a certain amount of individual attention and stimulation in order to develop her full potential. Parents of big families often just don't have the time to supply this. As a result, the children may not do as well in life as those from smaller families with more time and resources.

In the past, all this meant that life could be very hard indeed. Women often died in childbirth, or died very young because of the stresses and strains of poverty and parenthood. Many babies died at birth, and many children died very young through illness, disease or starvation. Parents had to face the prospect of losing most of their children before they grew up. Of course, it wasn't just contraception that changed this terrible state of affairs. Improvements in public health, proper sewers, clean water supplies and advances in medicine all played their part. But smaller families through choice have contributed, even if just by making it possible for us to control the quality of our lives.

Our freedom to choose parenthood means that we can now make a conscious decision. We can say things like "Yes, I want to have a baby, but not yet. Not until I'm ready." That sort of decision implies having reasons. This chapter is about the sort of reasons which will make the experience of becoming a parent as good as it can be, if that's what you decide to do.

Happy families

One friend of mine was very surprised when she heard me talking about having reasons for becoming a parent. "You don't need a reason," she said. "It's just part of a natural progression. You're born, you grow up, you get married and have your kids. Everybody does it."

That is one way of looking at it, I suppose, but not one which appeals to me very much. It's true that a lot of people *expect* you to become a parent just because everyone else seems to do it. But a lot of people expect you to do a lot of things, like wear a certain style of clothes or have your hair cut in a certain way. That's no reason to go along with their wishes.

Many of my friends said that almost as soon as they got engaged or married – or even started going out with someone regularly – their parents began to drop hints about 'the patter of tiny feet'. Some parents put enormous pressure on their children, daughters in particular, to start having babies. It's understandable, in a way; they may simply want to see their children going through the same process they did, assuming that it's inevitable. Some parents want their children to have the same pleasures that they got out of having *them*. You need to be aware of this sort of subtle pressure. It's your decision, and yours alone. In the end, you're the only person who knows when – or even if – you want to have children.

The pressures can come from further afield, too. Society in general tends to assume that all its members will want to do much the same things, and for most of us that means getting married and having babies. It can also mean, for women, that they are put under pressure to give up work to stay at home and look after their children, or at the very least accept that their careers will never be as important to them as they are to men. To men, it can mean missing out on much of their children's lives because they're expected to devote their time and energy to their jobs.

In fact you hear an awful lot of talk about 'the family' and how important it is. Everywhere you look you're surrounded by images of happy couples with their children (usually two, a boy and a girl). Newspaper and magazine advertisements and television commercials are full of happy families. It's almost as if everybody is telling you that it's not only *normal* to have children, it's absolutely necessary, and that if you don't want to be like everybody else there must be something very peculiar about you.

The result of all this pressure is that many of us find we're parents before we're ready. I have a feeling that Sally and I fell victim to this sort of thing; I know that once we were married our carelessness with contraception had a lot to do with thinking that as we were going to be parents anyway, we might as well get started. Although we love Emma, I think both of us would admit now that it would probably have been more sensible to wait a little longer. Financially Emma's birth was a disaster from which it took us several years to recover, and when I look at my monthly bank statements (they're like regular medical reports on a very sick relative) I sometimes wonder if we ever have – or will. I've lost count of the number of people I know who've said to me they wish they'd waited a little longer – 'until the time was right' – before becoming parents. The fact is that once you have a baby, you've got a responsibility. You're tied to that child and a certain way of life for the time it will take her to grow up and become independent. That means your options are limited and your freedom restricted. And however much they love their children, there isn't a parent alive who doesn't wish sometimes that they could have a little more freedom.

This is often more of a problem for girls than boys. Having a baby obviously affects women more than men in one way at least, the physical; women are the ones who carry the baby in their womb and give birth. But traditionally, women in almost all societies throughout the world have been expected to take the largest share in the burden of looking after and bringing up the children. Girls have always been brought up to see one of the main goals – if not *the* main goal – in their lives as being marriage and full-time motherhood.

Our society is still riddled with that idea, even today. Research in recent years has shown that parents still unconsciously influence their sons and daughters to behave and think about themselves and their futures in very different ways. Put bluntly, girls are given dolls and aprons to play with from an early age, while boys get toy soldiers, construction sets or spaceman suits. You can see it every day, all around you; little girls imitating their mothers by pushing toy prams, while their brothers play soldiers or going off to work, like daddy. I must confess that even my own two daughters, whose father is concerned about such things, much prefer to play with dolls than toy cars.

In that sense, girls' choices are often restricted. Many girls grow up thinking just like my friend, that becoming a mother is part of a 'natural progression' they can't – and don't want to – avoid. However, I'm hoping that even though my daughters like playing with their dolls, they'll realise when they're older that they don't have to follow the traditional woman's way – that they have a choice. Obviously enough, times have changed for women. The women's movement of the last twenty odd years has meant that women have more equality, greater opportunities and more choice in many areas of life – although there's still an awfully long way to go.

That's why it's important for more girls to realise they do have a choice. Women who give up all thoughts of a career and simply let themselves be swept along into motherhood often find that in later years they have many regrets. They won't be mothers all their lives; one day, their children will leave home and they'll have to find some point to life other than simply being a parent. If they have nothing to fall back on, life can suddenly become very difficult. Many women begin to feel something of this even while their children are still on their hands; but when you're in the full flow of parenthood, changing tack can be a very difficult business.

Later on in this book I'll be talking about alternative ways of life, of ways in which women can combine motherhood and a career or some other form of fulfilling activity. I'll also be talking about how these changes in women's attitudes to parenthood and their lives affect their male partners. Many men are turning away from traditional concepts of fatherhood which set them apart as breadwinners, and give them little contact with their families. I'm one of those men; and I'd like to take a bigger share in bringing up our children. I'd like to see more of them and more of my wife; but I've got a full time job, certain financial commitments (those bank statements!) and Sally hasn't had a job outside the home for many years, which means she would probably find it quite hard to get one now which paid enough to allow me to work less. So our room to manoeuvre is very limited indeed.

This is the point. If you're interested in doing things differently, then you need to start thinking about your options *before* it comes to the time when they are restricted. If you want to have children *and* a career, it needs organisation. The time to start making sure you get what you want is *now*.

Of course one of the major aspects of all this is money, which is the root of all evil, as we all know. Having a baby costs money. A recent survey put the cost of having a first child and bringing her up to the age of sixteen at £70,000! In Britain, medical care is free, but in other countries it may have to be paid for, and this can make the actual process of being pregnant and giving birth very expensive indeed.

But the costs don't stop with the birth. Obviously, the baby has to be clothed and all the necessary equipment – like a pram, a cot and so on – also has to be bought. Manufacturers these days are very good at making you believe you need more in the way of baby equipment than you actually do, so it's very easy to over spend on these items. The baby's mother may give up going out to work for a short time or for many years to look after her child. That means she'll no longer be earning – a net loss to the family's income.

Children obviously won't earn any money to be brought into the household either; they'll need to be supported, though, and for a long time. In simple terms, they cost more as they grow older. As babies they need food and warmth, love and security; and the only thing which doesn't have to be paid for out of those is the love. As they get bigger their needs – and therefore the costs of looking after them – grow in proportion. Don't forget that you will have to buy everything your child needs until he reaches adulthood – food, clothes, shoes, books and so on. Remember too that many couples decide to move to a bigger house with a garden when they start a family, and buying a house is probably the most expensive thing anyone can do in their lives.

The plain fact is, therefore, that a major problem for most young families is simply not having enough money. I know that most of my friends with children are, like me, chronically short of cash. Worrying about money can put a strain on your health and your relationships. It's often very hard on young fathers, who find themselves working long hours at a time when they would prefer to be at home with their families.

In simple terms, the more financially secure you are, the less troublesome parenthood is likely to be. I know that sounds unfair, almost as if I'm saying that you have to be rich to become parents. That's patently untrue. But take it from me, not having any money can spoil life with a baby – just having enough to get by can make all the difference.

Research has shown that it's the couples who really have to struggle on very low incomes who are the ones likely to face more problems. These difficulties range from health problems to straightforward financial ones, from not being able to afford to eat a proper diet of good foods, to living in very bad housing. It's that old link between poverty and children again – even today, babies can keep you poor and make you very unhappy, especially if you start off at a disadvantage. That's why if you can, it might be better to wait until life is more settled and prosperous.

So why have a baby?

Even though people haven't always had the choice, they've still generally given reasons for wanting to have children. Many people, for example, simply believe that it *is* a natural thing to do, and for them that's good enough.

Another common reason which you still hear today is that having children is a way of leaving something of yourself behind after you die. In a sense, you could see it as the easiest means – perhaps the *only* means – of gaining some form of immortality; in your children you can live forever.

It's true that most children outlive their parents, and that they in their turn are likely to have children of their own. Those children themselves will probably have children, and so on, into the infinite future. Part of this for some people is a desire to keep their own family name and traditions going. Some simply want to have children who will inherit their money or property.

But the child you create isn't *you* – she's a completely new person made from you and your partner. Of course, half of that child comes from you, and she will inherit some of the way you look, some of your personality. We all know that some children look very much like one or other of their parents. But that child's children will only inherit a quarter of their bodies and personalities from their grandparents, in the genes which are handed on to them; and *their* children only an eighth. Within a few generations, very little of what you've passed on to your children will remain; and very few of us even know anything about our great, great grandparents, without thinking of going any further back.

Other people I've talked to said that their decision to have children was influenced by their own family experience. Most of us have some memories of our own childhoods, whether happy or unhappy. Some people say that their childhoods were so happy they want to re-create them by becoming parents; they can then give a new generation of children the chance to have the same sort of happiness. Oddly enough, still others said it was because their own childhoods were unhappy, or their relationships with their parents went wrong in some way, that they wanted to have children to see if they could do it differently.

Linked to this is the desire to have someone to love, and who will love you. Those of us unlucky enough to have had unhappy childhoods sometimes grow up with a real need for love, and from the outside, it looks as if the relationship between parent and child is guaranteed to provide that, at the very least. Some people are also afraid of being alone and lonely in their old age, with no one to look after them, no fulfilment as grandparents. Others simply don't want to miss out on an experience that many people have, thinking that they'll always wonder what it would have been like if they don't do it.

None of these alone, seem like good reasons to me. First, there's no guarantee that you and your children will give each other the sort of love you might think you need. Most people *do* love their children much of the time; but children can be quite incredibly unlovable. I also think it's wrong to expect your children to be a prop to you in your old age; by that time they'll almost certainly have their own lives to lead, with families of their own, or careers, or both. I believe that good as it is to have a family, each member of it should be – as far as possible – independent and self supporting. And as for being worried about missing out on an experience – there are many, many things most of us never do, without regretting it. So why should *not* having children be all that different?

Perhaps the worst – and most worrying – reason of all for having children is plain, old fashioned romanticism. This is often the product of those pressures in society I was talking about earlier, and also that 'conspiracy of silence' about the bad things in parenthood. It's also why I'm writing this book. I've met many people who have a very rosy, idealised picture of parenthood and children. To them it all looks like sweetness and light and love. Of course being a parent is a wonderful experience in many ways, one which includes lots of love and pleasure and satisfaction. But it is also hard work, it's tiring and frustrating and sometimes full of problems.

Of course, if you start out thinking that everything is going to be perfect, the real thing will come as something of a shock. It's been shown in several research studies that the more romantic your vision of what parenthood is about, the harder you'll actually find it in practice. Some young mothers suffer from depression, and one factor which plays a part in it is the shock and disappointment of finding out that life with a baby often isn't very rosy after all.

Mixed reasons

Most of the parents I know would admit that their own reasons for having a baby are quite complicated, and probably a mixture of some of those I've discussed, plus a few other, more personal ones. Some of them would also say that if they'd known what they were letting themselves in for, they would have thought about it a lot more beforehand.

In fact, as you can see, many of the reasons I've put forward in this chapter for *having* children could also be taken as reasons *not* to. But there are others, too — and better ones. Before we look at them, though, it has to be said that one very large element in anyone's 'decision' to bring a new human being into the world is that instinctive, biological urge I talked about at the beginning of this chapter. It is very, very powerful; any woman who has felt 'broody' over a baby will testify to that, and even men get the same feeling sometimes — though not usually until they're already fathers. Like love and sex — with which it's linked — it's an instinct which can sweep you away without you even knowing.

Even so, I can't emphasise enough that you do have a choice. Try to remember one very simple thing. Three people are involved in making a baby; a man, a woman and the baby herself. Two of those three people have a choice about what they're doing; the third doesn't. Nobody asks to be brought into the world, and that makes it our responsibility to make sure we're doing the right thing — and at the right time — for all concerned.

That leads me to what I think are the best reasons for having a baby. They're very simple. The first is based on that idea of making every child a wanted child. If you know you *want* to have a baby – that is, you know you want to create a new, unique human being – then you really should be off to a flying start, so long as you also know something of what you're letting yourself in for. That means you have to be ready to go through all the things I'm going to describe in the rest of this book. Ready to go through pregnancy and childbirth, ready to accept the changes and challenges and to try and cope with them. I'll be saying further on a lot about how you shouldn't expect to cope on your own all the time; but the main burden must fall on a baby's parents, they have the final responsibility, and they're the ones who are going to have to cope.

Connected to this is another reason, and one which I've heard many people talk about. That's the desire to have a baby with a particular person, someone you love. This can be a powerful motive, and it's got a lot to do with the decisions people make to live together or to get married. It's difficult to describe, but from personal experience I know that having a baby is a way of making the love between two people grow. It takes a relationship to a new stage, and gives it a chance to change into something deeper and more rewarding. Again, it's important to remember that having a baby is something which can also damage a relationship, perhaps even drive a wedge between two people who love each other.

Friends without children have sometimes asked me how I could bring mine into a world like ours. "You only have to look at the newspapers or the television," one said. "Overpopulation, pollution, starvation – and we're all facing the prospect of nuclear annihilation. Why bring more innocents into the world to suffer?" I had to admit that my friend had a good point, and I do worry about my children's future a great deal.

But having children can bring many rewards, too. It must, otherwise people wouldn't do it – biology notwithstanding. Those rewards plug you into some of the best things in the human race; children are a new start, an expression of hope that the future can be different, better. They can be an expression of love and the stimulus to their parents to live a wider, fuller, richer life. That's what this book is all about; if it helps you to get those things out of having your own children, then I'll be happy.

Keeping your freedom to choose

Everyone has the right to make their own decisions, especially where it involves something as important as having a baby. In the end, only *you* can know whether you want children or not, or when the time is right.

But even in these days of widespread contraception, many people let their freedom to choose slip away. In Britain, for example, though contraception is very widely available and most schools have sex education classes, the number of teenage girls who become pregnant outside marriage is actually rising slightly, and has been since 1977. In a survey quoted in *The Guardian*, it was found that nearly 50 out of every 1000 girls between the ages of fifteen and nineteen in Britain became pregnant in 1980. Of those, 30 had their babies, and the rest had abortions. Girls even younger than that also became pregnant; some as young as twelve or thirteen.

Even though attitudes are much more relaxed about pregnancy outside marriage, becoming pregnant by accident can still be a catastrophe. I said that our first daughter was something of a mistake; but we were in our twenties, we already had somewhere to live (even though it wasn't ideal), and we were committed to the idea of becoming parents anyway. Even so, life was hard for a while. For a fifteen year old girl who is still living at home, a pregnancy can have a devastating effect on her life.

If you became pregnant at a similar age, you'd have to start making some pretty big decisions. If you decided to keep the baby – and your parents were supportive – you would still find it infinitely harder to study and get the qualifications you need to find the job you want. And we all know that finding any job is getting harder and harder these days. You and the child you have will need to be supported financially, and although your parents will probably want to help, they might simply not be able to. Remember too that you will have to take your child into consideration in every decision you take for years to come.

Many women – even quite young women – are deciding to keep their babies and to try and make a go of it as single parents. They might be forced into this sort of decision if their parents don't want to – or can't – help them and none of the other alternatives are suitable. Many single parents manage marvellously; but it has to be said that life for them is very difficult. Single parents have to support themselves if they can, and that means they have to find someone to look after the baby while they're out to work.

There are other alternatives. You could have your child adopted, although that's not always as easy as it sounds. Plenty of people are willing to give children a home. But many women who have their babies adopted feel very guilty about it. Some even spend the rest of their lives wondering if they've done the right thing, where their child is, how she is and whether she's being treated properly. In any case it still means you've got to go through pregnancy and birth only to hand your child over to someone else afterwards. That's often more difficult than it might sound – and it can be very, very upsetting.

In many countries abortion is available – that is, you can have your pregnancy ended medically. In early pregnancy it's quite a straightforward, simple procedure in which the womb is literally cleared out, either by suction or with instruments. The woman is under anaesthetic. In later pregnancy, though, it's done by actually stimulating the body to give birth, and it can be a very distressing experience. In most countries it's illegal after around the 26th week of pregnancy – the time at which the baby is considered to be 'viable'.

Abortions aren't always that easy to come by though, especially in countries where they're banned for religious reasons. The Catholic church is opposed to abortions, as are many other groups and organisations. In Britain, the legal age of consent to sexual intercourse is sixteen, so if you're under that and pregnant, you and the boy or man involved, may well come into conflict with the law.

But again, whatever you believe about the rights and wrongs of abortions, feelings have to be taken into account as well. Some women who've had abortions also feel very guilty about it afterwards, and the guilt can lead to depression. They wonder whether they've done the right thing, and what the child would have been like if she had been born. However well the rest of your life turns out, that abortion may stay in your memory.

This book is not the place to enter into a discussion on the rights and wrongs of abortion or the religious question. Some may disagree but having a pregnancy terminated may well be a better alternative than an adoption, or rushing into marriage. That, of course, is the traditional way of dealing with an unwanted pregnancy – a 'shotgun wedding', with the young couple forced to marry to make sure the child isn't illegitimate. I recently came across a fascinating statistic which shows just how strong this idea still is. In one in four marriages in Britain, the girl is pregnant – and the younger the bride, the more likely she is to be expecting a baby.

Many young couples find themselves pressured into getting married when the girl becomes pregnant. To their parents and society in general it might seem like a good idea. But it certainly isn't a good start to married life. The divorce statistics show that these are the marriages most likely to break up, and divorce can be a very upsetting experience for all concerned – not least the children.

Other statistics reveal some more equally worrying facts. Young couples who start off in this way, unprepared for marriage or parenthood, tend to have financial problems. They're also more likely to have difficult pregnancies, difficult births and children with more problems than average, both in terms of behaviour and health. They have a greater chance of becoming involved in family violence too – and it's all because they're under so much pressure. So you can see that one wrong turning early in life can have very large consequences.

Let's not forget the fathers of unwanted children, either, in this context. They too may well feel guilty if the girls they've got pregnant have an abortion or the child is adopted, and men also are sometimes prey to depression and upsets over adopted children. Other young men find themselves in a marriage they don't want or supporting a child financially for many years, something which can make life very hard.

So an unwanted pregnancy can cause great suffering all round, whatever the outcome. That's why it's so important to understand and use methods of contraception when you start having a sexual relationship, whenever that might be. If you're under age, getting hold of contraceptives can be difficult; which is a good reason for waiting before you start to have sex. It's always a good idea to wait before taking any big step in life. If you do take that step, effective contraception is the only means you have to protect your freedom to choose how you live your life. If you want to know more about the methods of contraception ask your doctor, who may be able to help you himself or send you on to a clinic which specialises in family planning.

Choices follow choices

If you *do* decide to have a baby, the decisions and choices you'll have to make won't end there. That's part of the reason why it's such a big change; it's just the beginning of a whole series of decisions you're going to have to make. In a way, that first decision to get pregnant is 'pregnant' with all the other decisions which have to come after.

These are many and varied, and range from the very important to the very minor. For instance, during your pregnancy you're going to have to decide whether or not to take your doctor's advice on many things, whether you should go to antenatal classes or not, and what sort of birth you want for your child. All these things are up to you – and it's important for you to bear that in mind. You're also going to have to decide things like what name to give your child (the name she's going to be lumbered with for the rest of her life).

There will be plenty of people around you throughout her life to help and advise, and you should use their support. But for many years to come you'll be completely responsible for the new human being you decide to create. You have the power to create life; that power entails responsibility. And the best place to start exercising that responsibility is in your own health.

3. Healthy parents, healthy babies

ONE OF THE FIRST questions most people ask about having a baby is "How do I make sure that everything goes well and that my baby is born healthy?" The answer – at least in most cases – is very straightforward. Your chances of having a trouble-free pregnancy, an easy birth and a healthy baby are all improved if you're healthy and fit to start with.

Before we can look at how you can make sure you are, we need to define exactly what 'health' is. In very simple terms, most doctors would say that your health depends on your whole self and your way of life. It depends, of course, on the state of your body, but that's something which is determined by – and linked with – many things. How happy and relaxed you are – or aren't, as the case may be – influences your health, as does the amount of stress in your life. Where you live, what job you do, the material conditions of life are important too. The sort of constitution you've inherited from your parents is part of the picture – and of course whether you smoke or drink alcohol or take any harmful drugs also has a great effect. And last but not least, doctors are now increasingly convinced that the sort of food you eat has an enormous influence on both the short and long term state of your health.

In short, our health is determined by the sort of people we are and the lives we lead. This might not sound very important, but it is – for doctors are now saying that the way many of us live in the developed, industrialised countries is simply not good for our health. For example, heart disease is now one of the biggest killer illnesses in all the rich countries of the world. Every year it causes hundreds of thousands – perhaps even millions – of people to die before they should. Doctors are now almost certain that most cases of heart disease are caused by things characteristic of our societies – smoking, eating the wrong sorts of foods and a lack of exercise.

3. Healthy parents, healthy babies

Some forms of cancer have also been linked with poor diet as well as smoking.

I've got two important points to make at this stage. The first is that it's never too late to start getting healthy. You might discover after reading this chapter that you've been doing the wrong things for years. But you'll start to feel the benefits as soon as you make changes. Even if you wait until you become pregnant before you give up smoking or change your diet, you and your baby will still be better off – so long as you do these things.

The second point is that by making yourself fitter and healthier, you'll not only be better able to cope with the stresses and strains of pregnancy and birth, you'll also be able to cope with life as a parent more efficiently. If you can make sure you start parenthood as fit and as stable as possible, you'll be doing yourself – and your children – a favour. Remember that what follows applies to men as well. Children deserve happy, healthy fathers too!

Those of us who live in the developed countries have a wider choice in what we eat than almost any other people in the history of the human race. Take a look round any supermarket and you'll see that there's a vast range of food available. It comes from all over the world, and much of it is processed and packaged to make life easy for us.

These mountains of food create all sorts of problems. One which is very obvious is that having an abundance of food leads to lots of people being overweight. Fatness, to put it bluntly, kills; it puts a strain on the heart and circulation for a start, and doctors now say that the fatter you are the more likely you are to die of a heart attack or stroke.

But the problem goes deeper than that. Much of the food we eat has had its natural goodness removed by processing. That's why many chemicals are added to foods, as well as substances to add colour or flavour. All these things can make food harmful to us.

We also eat a lot of junk food; chips, crisps, hamburgers, sweets, cakes, chocolates, fizzy drinks. Those foods which contain a lot of fat – things like fried chips and crisps, for example – are extremely bad for you if they form a large part of your diet over a long period of time. That's because too much fat in your diet can increase your chances of having heart disease, heart attacks or a stroke. In general, frying anything will make it more fatty. Some doctors would also say that we eat too much fatty meat, as well.

Sweets and cakes are full of sugar, and that's a substance which has one very direct effect; too much of it can rot your teeth. But sugar is also increasingly named as a contributory factor in a lot of illnesses, such as heart disease and bowel problems. Refined white sugar has been linked with diabetes. And of course, sweet, sugary foods are prime causes of the disease which some doctors call the most common illness of the twentieth century, at least in the developed countries – fatness.

Something which we need in our diets – and which many of us don't get, or at least not enough – is *fibre* or *roughage*. This is the indigestible part of foods like vegetables and grains, and it has one very useful quality; it helps your bowels to work smoothly. In simple terms, it doesn't get broken down in your gut, so as it passes through it keeps everything moving.

Again, it's the processing of our food which tends to take out the fibre. Take bread, for example. Wholemeal bread has plenty of fibre because it's made from the whole grain, and therefore includes the *bran*, or fibre part of the grain. White bread is made from white flour – which has had all the bran removed. Tinned and processed vegetables lose most of their fibre, as do vegetables which are cooked too much.

The first thing that a lack of fibre will do to you is to give you constipation. If this continues – and you have to strain each time you go to the toilet – you'll probably end up with *haemorrhoids*, otherwise known as *piles*. These are, quite simply, varicose veins of the anus. All that straining may also lead to straightforward varicose veins in the legs. Some doctors think that a diet without enough fibre will also make you want to eat a lot of starchy and sugary foods, which are fattening and bad for you.

So as you see, much of our ill health starts with what we eat. No one's saying that the odd bar of chocolate or hamburger is going to mean you'll be unhealthy, have heart disease or give birth to a handicapped child. But it's a fact with lots of evidence to back it up that *you are what you eat.*

A balanced diet

So what are the ingredients of a balanced diet? You can see that it's important to eat only natural, unprocessed foods as far as possible. A balanced diet contains certain essential things. these are protein, carbohydrates, vitamins, minerals, fibre and fat. If you eat foods which give you all of these in the right proportions, then you won't go far wrong.

Proteins These are the building blocks of your body, which uses them to make cells wherever they are needed. You can get protein from meat, fish, dairy products like milk and cheese, eggs, peas, beans, soya products and nuts. It's probably wise to keep your meat intake down, and to make sure that the meat you do eat isn't too fatty. Doctors these days also recommend that you shouldn't eat too many eggs, either, as they contain high levels of a substance called *cholesterol* which has been linked with heart disease.

Carbohydrates These provide your body with the energy it needs for all its activities, and they also help to build tissue. Carbohydrates come from bread, pasta, rice, all of which are also good sources of protein – if they're wholegrain. Sugar is another source of carbohydrates, but as you'll realise by now, this should be kept to a minimum in your diet – if not cut out altogether.

Vitamins Most of us know that vitamins are good for you. In fact they're substances we need to help keep vital processes in our bodies going. Shortages of vitamins can make you ill in various ways, and a severe deficiency can make you very ill indeed. For example, one of the B group of vitamins is called *folic acid*. This helps the body to make red blood cells, and a shortage of it can lead to *anaemia*; pregnant women are especially at risk. Folic acid is present in liver and fresh vegetables. Vitamin D is essential for our bones, and a shortage can lead to a disease called *rickets*; we get vitamin D from sunlight (which stimulates our skin to make it), oily fish, butter and eggs. Vitamin C is particularly important, too. It has a role to play in many areas, from breathing and growth to fighting off infection and stress. Vitamin C comes from fresh vegetables and fruit, especially citrus fruits like oranges. Vitamin K is essential for the proper clotting of the blood, and therefore helps to ensure you don't die from a minor cut; it too is found in green leafy vegetables. I could go on through an enormous list of vitamins, many of which are connected in groups, like the B group. Few people these days suffer from a major deficiency, but many of us have minor shortages. Eating a balanced diet of natural foods should give you the right vitamins – but be careful that you don't lose them by overcooking.

Minerals The body needs many minerals, and they are just as important as vitamins. Calcium is a good example. You can get it from milk, vegetables and eggs, and it's used by your body to build and maintain healthy teeth and bones. Iron helps to stop you being anaemic, and you'll get that from green, leafy vegetables and liver. Minerals are found in most natural foods.

Fats A certain amount of fat is important in anyone's diet, but it's vital to keep in mind that you don't need too much. Animal products aren't the only sources of fat; wholewheat bread, nuts, vegetable oils, and vegetables can also supply you with fat, and they're probably much better for you than eating a lot of meat. Dairy products like milk, cheese, cream, butter and yogurt are also sources of fat – and that's why you need to be careful with them. Although a certain amount of milk is good for you, too much butter and cream isn't. Dairy products have also been linked with other problems like allergies.

Something else we tend to overdo in our diets is salt. Too much salt in our food over a long period of time can have an adverse effect on the blood pressure, and high blood pressure is a problem which is particularly bad for pregnant women. It's a dangerous condition anyway, possibly leading to heart problems and strokes in later life if nothing is done about it.

The dangers of slimming

Slimming can also be a problem in itself – if it's taken too far.

It is a fact that far too many people in our society are overweight. Those extra pounds do shorten people's lives because they're a strain on the heart, the lungs, the circulation. You can see just how much of a problem it is by the number of people making money out of it with slimming advice in books, magazines and television programmes.

But do you remember those advertisements I talked about in Chapter 2? The ones which portrayed all those happy families. Advertisements also have an effect on the way people think of beauty, and in simple terms, our society says – through its images – *thin is beautiful*.

All this puts a lot of pressure on girls. It's very easy to get worried that you're too fat, when anyone will tell you that you're not at all, or only a couple of pounds overweight at the most. We're all sensitive about our appearance; and the emphasis on slimness in our society can make us take slimming too far.

There's been a lot of talk in recent years about a condition called *anorexia nervosa*. This is slimming taken to a dangerous extreme. It's almost always girls who suffer from it; they become obsessed with their weight and appearance to such an extent that they virtually starve themselves. Some girls have reached the point of serious illness and have needed hospital treatment. Some have even starved themselves to death.

In these tragic cases, there's probably an emotional or psychological element which has made the problem worse. But our society's insistence on slimness must take some of the blame.

This sort of illness has a direct relevance to your chances of having a baby. Of course, going without nourishing food is going to affect your body as a whole; it makes you weaker, more prone to illnesses and infections. It will also affect your menstrual cycle, and therefore your fertility. Some girls with extreme anorexia nervosa stop having periods altogether. The other point to remember is that, with the hard work involved in being a parent, your body is going to need a few reserves to fall back on. So remember not to overdo the slimming!

Fit for life

Human beings have bodies, and our bodies are designed to be used. Even if you eat a perfectly balanced diet, you might still be overweight if you don't take enough exercise.

That doesn't mean you have to be ready to run the marathon. But one other problem of our society which doctors have highlighted as causing a lot of ill health is that we have a tendency to be lazy – that is, we don't use our bodies enough.

Our primitive ancestors, for instance, couldn't drive to the supermarket and use a shopping trolley to collect what they needed. They had to go out and look for their food. Much of the time they had to chase it, a very physical activity indeed. Over thousands of years our bodies developed to cope with that sort of life; now we use the car instead.

Many of us take little exercise; some of us take none at all. We drive instead of walk, we take lifts instead of climbing the stairs, we sit in armchairs watching sport on the television instead of going out to do some ourselves. An unused body becomes very unfit. Heart and blood circulation problems are the main, long term result, but in the short term, a lack of exercise means that even the slightest physical effort can be a real strain.

Being unfit also makes life difficult in other ways. It means you won't sleep as well as you would if you took regular exercise. Your bowels are likely to work more slowly. You'll feel generally more slow, and your brain will probably be a bit less sharp. All in all, you won't work as well in any department as you could do if you were fit. If you've been fit in the past and let it slip, you'll know how much of a difference regular exercise can make.

Exercise will also help to keep your weight down, and its main benefit in terms of having a a baby is that it will help to make pregnancy and childbirth easier. Remember that childbirth is an intensely physical activity; some women say it's the toughest physical exercise they've ever done in their lives. If you want to make it easy for yourself, it's a good idea to be as fit as you can – and fitness can begin years before you even get pregnant.

It's important for both parents to be fit, by the way. Look at all the things I've said being fit can do for you – isn't it just as important for a baby's dad to be healthy, sharp, full of energy and zip?

How you get fit is up to you. We're lucky to live in a time when sport and getting fit has become enormously popular. There's a huge range of activities which you can get involved in: dance, walking or jogging, cycling, exercise classes, swimming, squash, and all the traditional, organised team sports. Whether you want to exercise to a tape or video in your own home, play football or go jogging, it's all out there just waiting for you to join up. And by doing so you'll make life healthier for your baby – from the start.

Smoking and drinking

There can be few people today who don't know that smoking can seriously damage your health. I recently watched a television programme in which a doctor said that out of 200 people he had treated for lung cancer – they all died – 198 were, or had been at one time, smokers. The other two, he added, had worked in very smoky environments for many years.

It's been proved that smoking does kill, by lung cancer or by heart disease, or by several other illnesses which have all been linked to cigarettes. Smoking is also a very expensive habit, and one which, while it's killing you, will make your clothes and hair smell, stain your teeth, and lower your resistance to infection. Every year, millions of working days are lost because smokers come down with cold after cold which develop into bronchitis.

If you detect a note of real feeling about this, you'd be right. It's the dedication of the convert, for I am one of the millions of people who in recent years have given up smoking. It's been hard; I would be dishonest to say it hasn't. That's why it's so important that you should never start, for physical addiction to any drug – and that's what addiction to cigarettes is – is always difficult to break. But if you are a smoker, try to give it up, especially if you're thinking of having a baby.

Women who smoke during their pregnancy can damage their children's health while they're still in the womb. It's been found that smoking is related to lower birth weight in babies, and smaller babies often have more problems.

Children of mothers who smoked while they were pregnant have also been found to develop more slowly; some have been found to lag behind in their reading, for example. So remember that if you smoke while you're expecting a baby, you're forcing her to smoke too. You'll be starving her of oxygen and damaging her health before she's even born.

If you continue to smoke after your baby is born – and this applies to both parents – you'll continue to damage your children's health. Remember those statistics I quoted? The two people the doctor was talking about who hadn't been smokers; they'd just breathed other people's secondhand smoke. If you smoke near your children, they'll be doing the same thing. It's been proved that children whose parents smoke have more coughs, colds and bronchitis than children of parents who don't.

Alcohol is another problem in our society, and if you think it isn't, then you should keep in mind that in Britain, for example, one in 100 people is an alcoholic. That means they're dependent on alcohol, physically addicted to it to the extent that it damages their health – and probably ruins their family life, too. Most of us believe that the odd drink from time to time isn't going to do us any harm. That may be true, but many alcoholics felt the same way when they started drinking. It's important to remember that alcohol can be a very dangerous substance, mostly because it's so easily available.

Doctors also say that you don't have to drink excessively for alcohol to harm you. In most of its forms, it's pretty potent stuff, and a lifetime of steady drinking at even quite a low level is going to have some adverse effects on your brain, your heart and your stomach. The more you drink, of course, the bigger the effect on your health. There's a growing recognition in many countries that alcoholism is a very widespread problem indeed, and there are more sources of help and support for people who suffer from it; *Alcoholics Anonymous* is the best known organisation, with branches all over the world.

It's known now that alcohol can have a harmful effect on babies in the womb. Babies born to women who have drunk

3. Healthy parents, healthy babies

heavily through pregnancy also tend to be smaller at birth, and slower in their development, as well as having other problems. Doctors say, however, that a baby in the womb can be affected by even quite small amounts of alcohol – and so they recommend that you keep any drinking in pregnancy down to an absolute minimum, if you can't cut it out entirely.

Nicotine and alcohol aren't the only two substances you can take into your body. Our society is different from almost all the others which have gone before because of the range of drugs which are available to us.

In fact, future historians may well look back and say this was the age of drugs, so many different types are there.

There are drugs which you can buy directly from a chemist's or pharmacy, like Aspirin; and there are drugs for which you have to have a doctor's prescription. Many doctors – and other people too – say that we take far too many pills and tablets, and that this is dangerous. Drugs sometimes react with other drugs in our system, and it's only common sense to keep to a minimum the number of substances you take into your body.

Of course some people use drugs in a very different way. Most of us know something about drug addiction, and associate it with crime. Drugs like heroin are very addictive, and have a dreadful effect on the addict's health. But people also get addicted to some types of tranquillisers, so it's important to be careful about anything you take.

It's vital not to take any drugs or over-the-counter medicines during pregnancy unless it's absolutely unavoidable – and even then, you should only do so with your doctor's knowledge and under his direction. That's because the growing baby in the womb can be severely damaged by drugs. Women in the 1960s who took the drug Thalidomide before or during their pregnancies gave birth to terribly handicapped babies, most of them with missing limbs. Babies born to drug addicts are usually addicted to the drug themselves, and very ill, and suffer greatly as they are weaned from the drug in their early days.

German measles

You may well have had German measles when you were a child – its more important sounding medical name is *rubella* – and if you did you'll probably have nothing to worry about. For German measles can have a catastrophic effect on a baby if her mother catches it while she's pregnant. Some babies born to mothers like this can be very severely handicapped, with their eyes, hearing and brains damaged.

To avoid this sort of problem, there has been a campaign in the United Kingdom since 1970 to vaccinate girls against German measles before they are likely to become pregnant. That means most girls in Britain are immunised at school when they are thirteen.

If you know you weren't immunised at school, and you think you have never had German measles, it's worth asking your doctor to give you a test to see if you're immune to it or not. If you're not, you'll be able to have the vaccination – and that will save you a lot of worry when you do become pregnant. Remember too that immunity may not last you a lifetime, so it's important to have it checked regularly.

If you're already pregnant, try not to worry. One of the first tests doctors give pregnant women is for immunity to German measles. If he discovers you're not immune, at least you'll know that you've got to be careful to avoid coming into any contact with the illness while you're pregnant. You can then make sure you have the vaccination after the birth, so that you'll be immune for any future pregnancies.

Stresses and strains

Stress is a normal part of most people's lives. We all have our worries; we all sometimes have to rush, to do too much. We all have arguments from time to time. It's how much stress we have to face – and how we learn to cope with it – that's important as far as the state of our health is concerned.

Many experts feel that there's too much stress in modern life. They say that the pace of everything is too fast, and that we expect ourselves to be able to cope with too much change, too much speed, too many problems and decisions. Stress has been linked with all sorts of physical illnesses, like heart problems, high blood pressure, and more minor – but very distressing – problems like headaches, insomnia, indigestion.

The problem is that we react to most stresses in the same way. Some doctors call it 'the fight or flight response'. Our remote ancestors' lives were much simpler than ours. The sorts of stress they had to face were straightforward; things like fierce animals threatening them. Their reaction to this sort of physical threat was either to fight it or to run away. Either way, their bodies got ready for physical action; the blood pressure went up, the heart beat faster, the muscles tensed. Physically we are the same as our ancestors – but our problems are more complex. Many of the things which threaten us are more abstract: Will I get that job? Does she love me any more? Where Am I going to get enough money to pay that bill? But our bodies respond in the same way, a physical way which is linked with emotions like worry or anxiety.

If the problem goes on for a long time, then our bodies might get into the habit of reacting in this way to every minor stress. In the long run this means we won't be able to handle problems or changes effectively – and also that our health will suffer.

In many ways, looking at stress sums up this whole chapter. That's because the most stressful events of life are usually the ones which involve change or disruption, such as the break up of a long relationship or changing your school or job. Probably the biggest change in anyone's life comes when you have your first baby. That makes it a very stressful event as well.

How you respond to that stress depends on the sort of habits you've developed in your life. One very important way of coping with it is relaxation. Everyone needs to be able to relax from time to time. We all need to get away from our worries and concerns, however temporarily. Relaxation doesn't just have to mean collapsing in front of the television, either, although if you're active otherwise, even that might do you good once in a while (but not too often!). Hobbies and sports which take you out of yourself – and perhaps give you exercise too – will also give you a way of letting off steam. People who relax in this way often find that they don't get so worked up and that stress is easier to deal with. Outdoor exercise in the fresh air and sun also has another bonus; the sunlight stimulates the body to make an important vitamin, vitamin D.

It's also important to get plenty of good, physical rest in the form of regular, refreshing sleep. Different people need different amounts of sleep, and their needs vary at different times of their lives. Only you know how much is good for you – but you'll see that if you do have a baby, you're going to be missing out on some sleep and generally having a tiring time. So make sure you get plenty of rest before it happens!

The links between stress and problems in pregnancy and childbirth are, in fact, very direct. Research studies have shown that women who are tense, under lots of pressure and unhappy during their pregnancies often have more difficult births and smaller babies than average. The babies are also more likely to have health problems. This doesn't mean that *any* stress, however minor, is going to have this sort of effect; the women who suffered in these ways had been under prolonged, intense pressure. But it shows just how important it is to keep stress out of your life, especially at such a crucial time.

A stable relationship

I talked in the last chapter about women who bring up children on their own, couples getting divorced, and so on. But it's still a fact that most children are born to couples who are married; nine out of ten people get married and have children. However much society has changed in recent years, it's still very much based on the idea of two people, a man and a woman, living together and having children.

It isn't absolutely necessary for every child to be brought up in the 'traditional' way, though, with Mum staying at home full-time and Dad going out to work. Dads can do it, just as anyone can who is committed enough to do it properly. But notice that key word – 'properly'; they must have the right sort of care. What I am saying is that children are very sensitive plants. They respond very quickly to the *wrong* sort of care; they respond very quickly to changes and problems in their environment. What this means is that they need a certain amount of stability in their lives. I'm not simply talking about material stability in terms of regular meals and a comfortable place to live, although that helps; I'm talking about *emotional* stability, too. They need to feel secure, wanted, valued – in a word, loved.

You may have heard talk about the effect of divorce on children. My parents were divorced when I was five, so I know something about that. It can have a very powerful effect on a child, and this is something doctors, social workers, teachers and many other 'professionals' are well aware of. The worst time for a child in a divorce is often the time of argument and uncertainty which precedes it, the time of bad atmosphere and emotional upset. Children get over it, given the right amount of love and security. I believe it's better for a child to live happily with one parent after a divorce and see the other than to live with two parents who hate each other.

What all of this means is that I believe you should take into account the 'health' and stability of the relationship you're involved in before you take the plunge into having children. I'm saying it in that way because for most of us that's the way it happens; we're already in a relationship before the decision to have children is made. I don't think marriage is the right thing for every relationship, although some people still believe it is, when it comes to having a baby. But I do believe that it's good for babies to have two people looking after them, a mother *and* a father, if it's at all possible. It's a very sensible, practical arrangement.

Problems in our relationships with other people – particularly people we're closely involved with – are major causes of stress in anyone's life. And as we know, stress is directly connected to health. In this context, bringing a baby into a unstable relationship is like putting dynamite in the basement of a house with shaky foundations – not a very good idea, to say the least. Couples sometimes have a baby as a way of trying to make a relationship work; needless to say, unless there was something going for that relationship in the first place, it's not much of a solution.

That's why the experts say that the best age to have a first baby is probably in your mid to late twenties. Physically you're probably at your most fertile and fittest in your late teens and early twenties. But those are the years when you're just starting out in life. You probably won't have settled into a career, or decided exactly what it is you want to do. Those are the years when most of us meet someone we start living with, or perhaps even marry, and when we haven't got much money. Having a baby in those circumstances is going to be a bigger strain on you than if you wait a little longer.

Medical check-ups

In the next chapter I'm going to explain a few things about genetics, which is the scientific name for the way in which we inherit characteristics from our forebears. Here all I want to say is that it is possible to inherit illnesses — sometimes quite serious ones — and to pass them on to your own children.

For example, people from Mediterranean countries like Greece, Turkey and Cyprus sometimes suffer from a blood disease called *thalassaemia* which can be passed on to their children. *Haemophilia* is another disease children can inherit from their parents; this is the disease which affected many of Queen Victoria's relatives, in which the blood doesn't clot properly. Someone who suffers from it can, quite literally, bleed to death from the tiniest cut.

The important thing to remember is that you don't have to suffer from one of these diseases to pass it on to your children. You can be what's called a *carrier*; that is, you can have the gene which will pass on the illness and which will be activated in your child given the right circumstances.

Obviously, it's better to avoid passing on a serious, inherited disease if you can. Passing it on knowingly means you could be condemning a child to a lot of suffering. That's why in some hospitals today there are specialist clinics and doctors trained to discover whether you are likely to pass on any diseases to your children. If you're worried about this problem, it's worth asking your doctor to refer you to one of these clinics for special testing if it's at all possible. The technique is called *genetic counselling*, and it's important for both partners to go along; this is because in many cases, inherited disease is caused by the mixing of genes rather than one gene alone from one individual partner.

Some experts are even recommending that young couples should go to their doctors before they plan to conceive a baby anyway. The idea is that you should have a thorough medical check up *before* you set about making a a baby to ensure that you have no health problems, on the grounds that two healthy adults are more likely to produce a healthy baby. At this check up you could be given advice about any aspect of your life style – from your diet to the sort of stresses there are in your life.

We'll also see in the next chapter that it takes a few weeks – perhaps even a couple of months – for a woman to be sure she's pregnant, and it's in the first few months of pregnancy that the baby is at her most vulnerable to outside influences. It's therefore important to make sure your health is good, and you're not doing anything to affect your baby, before you even get pregnant. This new approach to pregnancy health is called *pre-conceptual care*, and it's what this chapter has been all about. Indeed, it's what this book is all about, and the rest of it is designed to make sure your mental health stays good after you've had a baby by telling you all the things you need to know!

I've only been able to skim the surface of the subject of pre-conceptual care. It's now known that many, many things can affect your health, and new evidence is being turned up almost every day. Before we move on I'd like to make a couple of points. The first is that you should keep this all in perspective. I don't want you to panic because you prefer white bread, or think you don't take enough exercise; it's worth doing all the things I've suggested, but nobody can be perfect, after all. Problems are more likely to occur if you do too many of the bad things for too long. The second is that doctors are now advising couples who have been using the pill as their method of contraception to switch to another method for a short period – say, three to six months – before they start trying to make a baby. This is because the hormones in the pill need to be 'flushed out' of the woman's system, and allow her body to settle down into its natural rhythms before she embarks on a pregnancy.

Part 2. **From conception to birth**

4. Conception

THE CREATION of a new human being, your baby, starts in that most obvious of places, the sex organs. Men's sex organs consist of a penis and two testicles. Women's sex organs are the vagina, the womb, the Fallopian tubes and the ovaries. In simple terms, men produce sperms in their testicles and these are brought to the vagina by the penis in sexual intercourse; they then swim up through the womb and Fallopian tubes, to meet the egg travelling down, one of them fertilises it – and that's the beginning of life.

But the seeds of that life have a long history beforehand. Sperms are produced in vast numbers in the testicles, for example – millions at a time. Each sperm is about 0.05 millimetres long, and consists of a head, a neck and a long, thin tail; they look very much like tadpoles under the microscope. And just as in a tadpole, the tail is what provides the motive power for that long swim towards the egg. The sperms are made in the thousands of closely packed tubes inside the testicle called *seminiferous tubules*. From there they pass to a

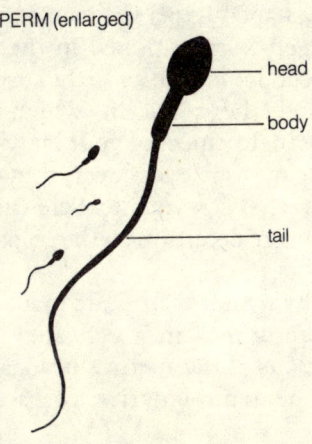

tube called the *epididymis*, then into another called the *vas deferens*. They then pass into the *seminal vesicles* where they are stored until they're needed in an ejaculation. A boy's testicles start producing sperms at puberty, and continue to do so almost throughout his life, although he may produce fewer and fewer (and of worse quality) as he gets older.

Interestingly enough, a girl is born with all the eggs or *ova* (singular, *ovum*) she'll ever need – and more than enough, in fact. She'll be born with about 80,000 immature eggs in her ovaries, of which she has two, one on either side of the womb. What happens to these is controlled by a tiny area of her brain called the *pituitary gland*. After she reaches puberty, each month this gland releases a special hormone which stimulates the ovaries to make yet another hormone, *oestrogen*, and also makes a number of the immature eggs develop. Out of these, only one becomes properly ripe. When it reaches this stage, it comes to the surface of the ovary, is released and picked up by the open, funnel-shaped end of the nearby Fallopian tube. This entire process – which is where we all started – is called *ovulation*.

So there they are – human sperms and eggs. But what's inside these seeds, these basic building blocks of human beings? In simple terms, each sperm and egg contains half of a blueprint for a person waiting to be matched by another half.

Our bodies are made of millions of cells, and each tiny cell contains 46 *chromosomes* arranged in 23 pairs. Each of those chromosomes is shaped like a little crossed rod, and clustered along it are the *genes* I mentioned in the last chapter which, under the microscope, look like little beads. These genes and chromosomes and the ways in which they are arranged determine every single aspect of your body – the way your nose looks, the colour of your eyes, everything. The last pair, the 23rd, determines what sex you are. Scientists now believe that your genes can even determine a large part of the way your personality turns out.

In the process by which sperms are made in a man's testicles, half of the chromosomes in a cell are shed. That cell then becomes the nucleus of the sperm's head, and only contains 23 chromosomes, one representative of each pair. A woman's eggs are made in much the same way, and they only contain 23 chromosomes, too. At the moment of conception, each chromosome finds a 'partner' and makes a pair. So eventually there are 23 pairs of chromosomes in a fertilised egg – 46 chromosomes in all, just as in the baby's mother and father.

We look like our parents because we get half of our genes from each of them; but we look uniquely like ourselves, not identical to anyone else, because the genes on our chromosomes combine in random, unpredictable ways. It is possible for very strong characteristics to dominate generation after generation of a family – like a 'family nose' – but it's also possible for one generation to look very different and not have that characteristic at all.

You might be wondering how it is that twins are possible if only one egg is released at ovulation. There are two types of twins; in one type, more than one egg is actually released and both (or more, if three, four or more eggs are involved) are fertilised, each by a separate sperm. This type is called *fraternal twins*. They resemble each other as much – or as little – as ordinary brothers and sisters, and it's just chance that they should be made at the same time.

The other type is called *identical twins*. These are the result of one egg being fertilised and then dividing into two completely separate cells soon after conception. Each of these cells then develops into a baby. They're called identical because that's what they are – they share the same chromosomes, so they are *exactly* alike.

Twins often run in families, and if they do in your family you have a higher chance of having twins yourself when you start to have children. In Britain your chances of having twins are about one in 80 – or one in 50 if you have a family where twins are quite common.

We've seen that everyone has 23 pairs of chromosomes, and that the last pair determine our sex. In females, that pair consists of two X chromosomes; in males, one is an X chromosome and the other is a Y. So when the pairs divide up to make eggs and sperms, two different things happen.

In women, because the last pair of chromosomes is XX, each egg has the same sex chromosome after division – an X. But

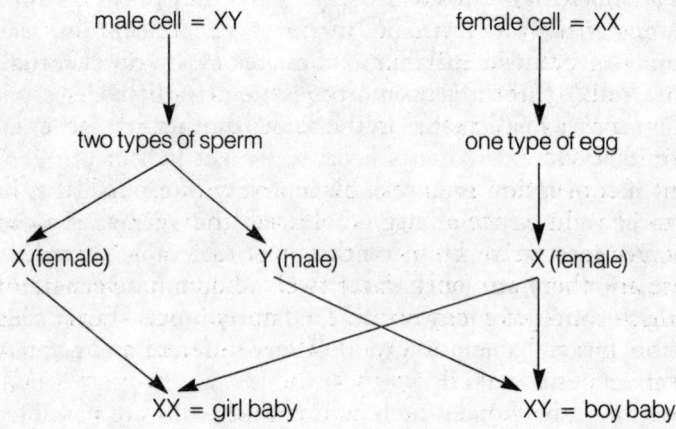

sperms can be either X sperms or Y sperms – that is, either female (X) or male (Y). This means that a baby's sex depends on what type of sperm fertilises the egg. If it's an X sperm, the resultant baby will be a girl, if it's a Y, the baby will be a boy.

The right time

Of course, the egg and the sperm still have to be brought together for a baby to be made. That's usually done through the medium of sexual intercourse. I say 'usually' because it has been known for a girl to get pregnant without actually having full intercourse. Sperms are very mobile – and they're very keen to achieve what they're designed to. If they're ejaculated on or near the outside of the vagina, they're perfectly capable of getting in and swimming up the Fallopian tubes – so you need to be careful.

At any rate, in sexual intercourse, the man's penis is placed inside the woman's vagina and *ejaculation* takes place. This is when the sperms, mixed with a special fluid called *semen*, which is secreted in the seminal vesicles and the prostate gland, are released into the vagina. There may be anything between 150 and 500 million sperms in an ejaculation – only one of which will eventually reach the egg and fertilise it.

Once they've been ejaculated into the vagina, the sperms

begin to swim up towards the *cervix* (the neck of the womb). Millions of them don't make it that far, and by the time the survivors reach the Fallopian tubes, a journey of about nine inches, only a few thousand will be left. It's thought that this is like a trial by strength; only the strongest and the fittest sperms survive.

But if conception is to take place, the timing of all this has got to be right. Once an egg is released from an ovary, it will only live for twelve hours at the most, unless it's fertilised. There are, therefore, only about twelve hours in every month in which conception can occur. That doesn't necessarily mean that sex has to happen at exactly the same time as ovulation. Sperms can survive for up to 48 hours in a woman's body, sometimes even longer. So if intercourse takes place a day or two before ovulation, there may still be enough sperms lurking around when the egg is released to ensure fertilisation. But a week before or after ovulation is obviously no use at all.

Ovulation isn't the only thing which happens in a woman's body under the stimulation of that hormone oestrogen (and another one called progesterone which is also produced in the same process). The lining of the womb – the *endometrium* – is stimulated to become thicker and more nutritious, for any egg which is fertilised will embed itself in the womb before it starts growing into a baby.

The cervix is also filled for most of a woman's cycle with a plug of mucus which makes it almost impenetrable to sperms. The hormones in the system at the time of ovulation make this mucus thinner and more watery – to help the sperms get through. Other changes take place as well, all with the purpose of making conception more likely.

If fertilisation doesn't take place, the egg dies and is absorbed into the body. The thicker lining of the womb is shed through the vagina, and that's what makes up the bleeding of a menstrual period. The level of hormones in your body drops, the mucus in the cervix thickens up, and the body waits for next month and another chance to get pregnant.

This process is called *the menstrual cycle*, and in most women it takes place every month from the time of their first period, their *menarche*, until the day they stop having periods altogether, the *menopause* (which usually happens in a woman's forties or, at the latest, her early fifties). Most women have a fairly regular cycle, and the average is about 28 days long, with the first day of your period counting as day 1 of your cycle. Ovulation, however, is always related to the period which follows, and this usually comes 14 days after the egg is released. So if you've got a 28-day cycle, you're likely to ovulate on the 14th day. If you've got a longer or shorter cycle, you're still likely to ovulate 14 days before your period.

Fertility problems

If you're a young healthy woman and you have intercourse fairly regularly for a year without using any form of contraception, you've got a 90 per cent chance of becoming pregnant within that time. In fact, doctors estimate that 25 per cent of couples who have decided to have a baby are successful in achieving conception within a month of starting to try. 80 per cent of couples manage to achieve a pregnancy within their first year of trying.

I've always found those figures quite surprising. You've seen in this chapter that the process of conception is a very complicated business, depending on many things for success. So it shouldn't be a shock to you to hear that some people experience a lot of difficulty in getting pregnant. These people are said to have *fertility problems*, and finding out that it's not so easy for *you* to have a baby as you might have thought can come as a terrible shock.

The causes of fertility problems are many and varied. Both men and women can have problems which can prevent them from having a baby. Some men, for example, don't produce enough sperms, or even any at all. There might be a blockage or a gap in one of the tubes leading from the testicles to the penis. Some women have blocked Fallopian tubes or hormone problems which mean they don't ovulate properly. The problem could actually be in something between the two partners; some women have *antibodies* in their system which attack and kill their husband's sperms as if they were invading germs.

Fortunately, doctors can now help very many couples who in the past would have been unable to have children. At the moment it's estimated that 60 per cent of couples with fertility problems can be helped to overcome them, and research is being carried out continually to increase that percentage. Indeed, it is research into infertility which has revealed many of the facts I've talked about in this chapter.

The treatments doctors can offer couples with fertility problems are as varied as the problems themselves. They range from hormone treatment to sort out a woman's periods – and therefore her ovulation – to full scale surgery to correct some sort of physical problem in the genital organs themselves. One of the most famous methods of treating infertility is the 'test tube baby' technique. This was developed to help women whose Fallopian tubes were damaged through infection to the extent that sperms or eggs couldn't pass through them and meet. The technique involves removing an egg from a woman's ovary by surgery, putting it into a dish with sperms from her partner and then replacing it in her body after it has been fertilised.

This 'last chance' treatment, which involves high technology and the fine skills of top surgeons, is probably the most expensive and complicated method of solving a fertility problem. For most women the answer could be much simpler. Making sure you have intercourse around the time of ovulation is probably the way of giving yourself the best chance of getting pregnant, and there are two other ways which doctors recommend to people to help them pinpoint the time of ovulation more exactly than just working it out in the woman's cycle. The first is that some women experience a pain in the lower abdomen when they ovulate. The second is that most women find their temperature goes up slightly when an egg is released. Keeping a daily temperature chart for a couple of months is the best way of making sure you pick up this rise.

Remember that it's important to seek help for difficulties with fertility before they've gone on too long. Some problems may take a long time to detect and solve. But it's also important not to panic if you don't get pregnant as quickly as you'd like. If your periods are irregular, you could check with your doctor; but you'll probably find, like most people, you'll have no problems.

New life is made

But let's get back to that moment when the sperm meets the egg. In fact, quite a few of the surviving sperms cluster round the egg when they come into contact with it. Only one will be able to penetrate it and achieve fertilisation, but that lone sperm needs the help of some of the other survivors. That's because a special substance is needed to turn the egg's outer covering into liquid for the sperm to enter. Each sperm carries a little of this substance, but no one sperm on its own has enough.

How that sperm makes its final entrance into the egg isn't known precisely. But once its head is through the outer covering, it sheds its tail, which is no longer necessary; the head of the sperm is where those vital chromosomes are, after all.

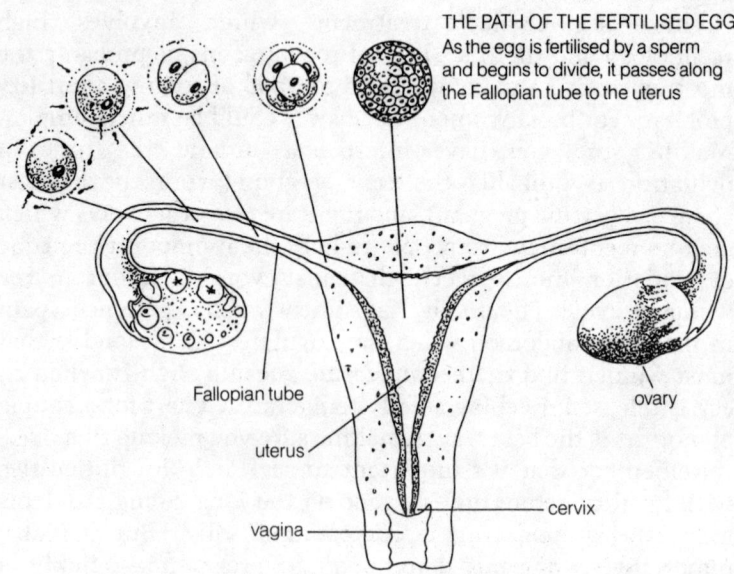

THE PATH OF THE FERTILISED EGG
As the egg is fertilised by a sperm and begins to divide, it passes along the Fallopian tube to the uterus

The egg contains its chromosomes inside a nucleus, and over a couple of hours after the sperm's penetration, these two collections of chromosomes expand and move towards each other. Finally they meet and fuse, and the chromosomes pair up, the genes combine – and new life has begun. The fertilised egg is now one cell with one nucleus containing a full blueprint for a new human being; a person who will be completely unique.

Very soon that cell divides into two. Each of these new cells contains a copy of that 46 chromosome blueprint. During the next three days, this new being continues to divide; first into four, then eight, then sixteen, then 32 cells and so on, each new cell containing an identical copy of that genetic blueprint. While this division has been going on, the fertilised egg continues to move down the Fallopian tube, and eventually it emerges into the womb. Between five and seven days after fertilisation it embeds itself into the wall of the womb, and the pregnancy has begun.

The first sign that a woman is pregnant is usually that she misses a period. In a woman with an average 28-day cycle, everything I've described has happened before she even has any reason to suspect that she might be pregnant; she hasn't even reached the time when she would normally expect her period.

Life in the womb

The average pregnancy lasts around nine months, or to be more precise, 280 days from the first day of the last period, or 266 days from conception itself. But it's the first three months or 90 days which are probably the most crucial time for the development of the baby. At the end of that time all the major organs are formed, and it's just a question of the baby getting mature enough to be born into the outside world.

At any rate, the first thing which has to happen once the fertilised egg – now a collection of cells in the process of division – has embedded itself in the womb is for the new *embryo* (as doctors call it) to make sure of its oxygen and food supply. This will come from the *placenta*, a piece of tissue on the side of the womb which develops from the embryo itself.

Blood from the mother arrives at the placenta and 'drops off' oxygen and nutrients to the baby's bloodstream, without the two ever coming into direct contact. The placenta is attached to the baby's stomach – at the navel – by the umbilical cord.

Part of the embryo also develops into a bag which surrounds the developing baby and placenta. This is called the *amniotic sac*, and it's filled with fluid. It's there to cushion the baby from any bumps or blows from the outside world, as well as for various other purposes.

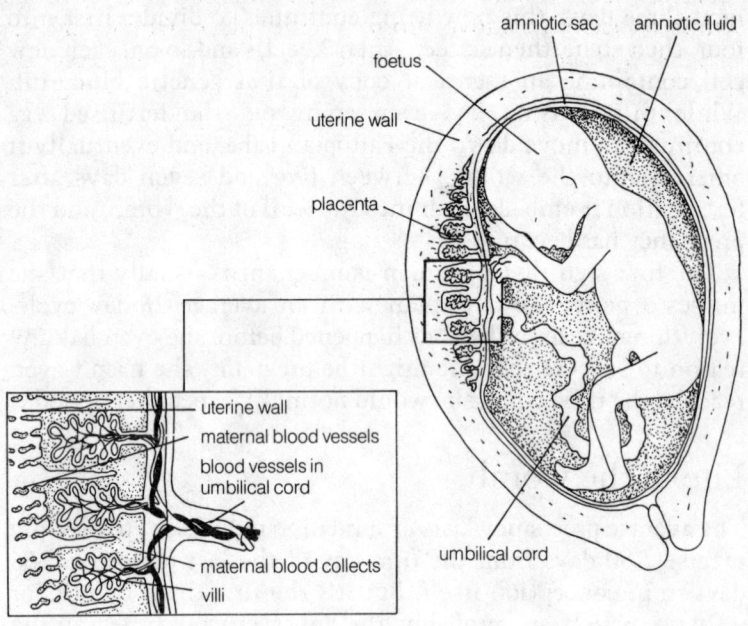

But, of course, the main thing that's happening inside the womb after conception is phenomenal growth and development. In the first month of pregnancy – before the mother is even aware that she's pregnant – her baby will develop from a single cell to a being with a recognisable head, a body and the beginnings of its internal organs. This embryo will increase in size during the same period 40 times over, and in weight 3000 fold. Seventeen or eighteen days after conception, the embryo has developed blood cells and the foundations of a heart. By about 20 days, the brain, spine and nervous system have begin to appear, and the eyes and ears start to develop as shallow depressions in the head. At about 24 days, the heart starts to pulse slowly. It won't stop moving for the rest of this new human being's life – perhaps for 70, 80 or even 90 years. By the fifth week, the embryo is big enough to be seen, and measures two millimetres long.

At about the same time, the embryo's sex organs begin to develop, too. Around the 21st day, a number of cells in the embryo begin to move along to the place where the sex organs will be. They are called *germ cells*, and once the testicles or ovaries begin to form, many of these cells stay inside them. Eventually, they'll turn into the raw material for the sperms or eggs which will go into creating this embryo's children.

By seven weeks, buds have begun to appear on the embryo, and these will eventually become the baby's arms and legs. The chest is properly formed, as is the intestine (almost), and the head is developing very quickly indeed. The face in fact forms itself by growing in towards the centre, the upper and lower jaws in particular coming together some time in the eighth week.

By week nine, the eyes are formed completely, but they're still covered by the skin which will eventually become the eyelids. A nose has appeared, as have rudimentary fingers and toes, and the foetus (as doctors call it by this stage) is even making some movements, although the mother won't be able to feel them for some time to come. By the tenth week the inner ear is formed, and the outer ear is beginning to appear.

By the eleventh week, all the major organs are formed; the heart is beating properly, the blood is circulating round the body, and it's possible to tell what sex the foetus is. Of course there is still much development to come, and organs like the lungs don't work properly yet. In fact, it won't be until later on in the pregnancy that many of the organs take on their proper functions; some don't even start working properly until the baby is born. But in all the essentials, the foetus is a recognisable, living human being at eleven weeks. By twelve weeks, this new person will be about 6.5 centimetres long – about the length of a bar of soap.

I talked in the last chapter about German measles having a devastating effect on a baby and causing severe handicap. This will only happen if a baby is exposed to German measles in the first three months of pregnancy. In fact because all the major organs are being formed at this time, the developing baby is vulnerable to all sorts of things – X-rays, drugs, infections like rubella. That's why it's vital for women who think they're pregnant to avoid anything which might be a risk to their babies. After the major organs are formed, there's a lot less chance of a baby being badly damaged by something – although you still need to be careful.

Growing to maturity

By the time she reaches the third month of her pregnancy, a woman is probably well aware that she's pregnant. By that time, too, her baby is a recognisable human being. A three-month-old foetus does look a little odd; the head is disproportionately large, the limbs are very skinny and the face looks a little bizarre. But everything is there. All that is needed now is time and the continuing nourishment and security of the womb for the job of growing to maturity to be finished properly.

At various times in the history of the human race it's been thought that nothing much other than physical development went on in the womb during pregnancy. In the eighteenth century, for example, before microscopes were invented, it was believed that sperms were actually complete little people (called *homunculi*), and that all the womb did was to provide nourishment and somewhere for the little person to grow into a baby.

We now know that a lot more than just growth goes on in the womb, although that's obviously important. Samuel Taylor Coleridge, the great English Romantic poet, once wrote something which has stuck in my mind ever since I first came across it: 'The history of man for the nine months preceding his birth would probably be far more interesting and contain events of greater moment than all the three score and ten years that follow it.'

It has become increasingly obvious through research in recent years that babies in the womb are quite *responsive*. This is something that mothers have always known; I've already said that babies move in the womb, and these movements eventually become strong enough for the mother to feel them. The moment when the mother feels her baby move in the womb for the first time is called *quickening*. It usually happens between the eighteenth and the 22nd week. In a first pregnancy you're unlikely to recognise the feeling – which some mothers say is like 'butterflies in the tummy' – at first. But in a second or subsequent pregnancy you're likely to feel it earlier on, mostly because you'll know what the sensation is like and won't mistake it.

At any rate, the baby's movements will get more and more acrobatic as she grows. Some women are even kept awake at night by their baby's kicking. It's one way the baby has of communicating with the outside world. That's not as weird as it sounds, because the baby has some idea the outside world is there; the womb isn't a completely soundproof environment, and some light penetrates it, too.

Many mothers find, especially in later pregnancy, that their babies react strongly to loud or unpleasant sounds near the womb. It's been shown that making a loud, sudden noise very close to a pregnant woman's tummy will often make the baby 'jump' with surprise and fright. Babies in the womb also respond to music; it's been reported that they tend to enjoy the more soothing varieties of classical music rather than loud, heavy rock or punk for example. It's not completely dark in the womb, either. Strong light penetrates the skin, and it's likely that babies in the womb can distinguish between light and dark, or day and night. The light they see, which comes through the blood vessels surrounding them, is probably orange-red; and that might be why many adults find reddish, 'warm' lighting so comforting.

Don't forget that even at as early a stage as four months in the womb, most of the baby's 'working parts' are already formed. Her ears are beginning to work, as are her eyes; and she can suck her thumb, too. It's likely that babies start sucking their fingers and thumbs quite early on, but they have been observed doing it at four months. They've got good reason to do this throughout their time in the womb; it gives them plenty of practice in the technique of sucking on which they're going to be dependent for survival when they come out of the womb.

Babies have also been observed getting some other sorts of practice in the womb. I've already said that they're surrounded by fluid, and that they get all the oxygen they need from the placenta. But they actually practise breathing movements with their lungs by 'breathing in' some of the amniotic fluid which surrounds them. By doing this they're making sure that they'll know how to use their lungs properly at that crucial moment when they're going to have to use them for real – at birth. They don't choke because they're getting oxygen 'direct' through the umbilical cord.

You might be thinking that this is all very interesting – but so what? The point is that from a very early stage, a baby in the womb is a very sensitive, responsive creature. If you remember, I talked in Chapter 3 about how important it is to try and cut out as much stress from your life as possible when you're having a baby. Scientists are now beginning to believe that stress has a very direct, physical effect on babies.

One very interesting experiment demonstrated this quite clearly. It's now known that even without any external sounds, the womb is a very noisy place. The baby can hear her mother's heart beating quite loudly, and her stomach rumbling; they're not all that far away, after all. It's also been discovered that playing a recording of heartbeats and other 'body' sounds to newborn babies makes them calmer and happier if they're crying – but only if the heart beats are at the 'right' speed of around 80 beats per minute. This is what a mother's heart rate would be when she is calm. If a recording with a higher rate of heart beats is played to the newborn babies – say around 100 beats per minute – they become distressed and unhappy. A mother's heart would start to beat at that rate if she was engaged in some sort of heavy physical exertion or if she was upset or distressed about something, that is if she was under stress.

You can see now why a baby will have more problems if a mother is under long term stress. A baby in the womb is so intricately enmeshed in the physical processes around her that she's probably highly sensitive to all sorts of changes which we don't notice at all, things like a sudden change in heart rate. Stress on a mother can stimulate the release of hormones like adrenalin into her blood, the hormone which prepares us for action when we're in danger; stress can make the blood pressure go up and the heart race. Her baby probably reacts to all this.

The last lap

At 28 weeks, the baby is said to have reached the stage where she is *viable*, at least according to the law in Britain. What this means is that she is now considered to be capable of survival if birth should take place. Obviously, the longer the baby can stay in the womb the better, but 28-week-old babies, and even younger ones, have survived, and doctors are continually improving their skills in saving the lives of very small, very premature babies.

At 28 weeks, the average baby is about 37 centimetres long and weighs about two pounds. Between this time and the birth, she's likely to put on another five pounds and grow to a length of 50 to 53 centimetres. But there's also a tremendous surge in another, much more important, part of a human baby's development in this last lap – and that's in the brain.

The human brain (along with the human hand) is what makes people different from the rest of the animal kingdom. In comparison to other animals it's enormous in proportion to our size – and it's a very complex organ indeed. It's the origin of all the things we take for granted in mankind: civilisation, science, language, art, religion. Its beginnings lie in the earliest weeks of pregnancy, but in about the seventh month its development takes off. The front part of the brain, for instance – the part which controls all the 'higher' functions like speech and abstract thought – enlarges so much it covers the rest of the brain entirely.

It is at about this time too that the brain begins to develop the twists, curls and depressions all over its surface which give it its familiar look. These actually help to increase the surface of the brain which is available for use. However, scientists now think that few of us ever use the the full potential of our brains, and that even the cleverest of adults still has more brain 'capacity' than he or she uses. This has important implications which I'll be looking at in Chapter 8 when I come to look at child development. Here I'll say that it's the human baby's need for a long time to allow her brain to develop which makes human childhood longer than any other animal's – and that it's up to parents to help their children achieve the best possible use of their brains.

At any rate, it's interesting to note that researchers now think that babies in the womb begin to develop definite personalities of their own at about seven months, that is, at about the same time as their brains begin this surge of development. It's also thought that babies have dreams in the womb.

When we adults dream, our brains exhibit special wave patterns, and our eyes tend to move in rapid, jerky ways. That's why the type of sleep during which dreams occur is called REM

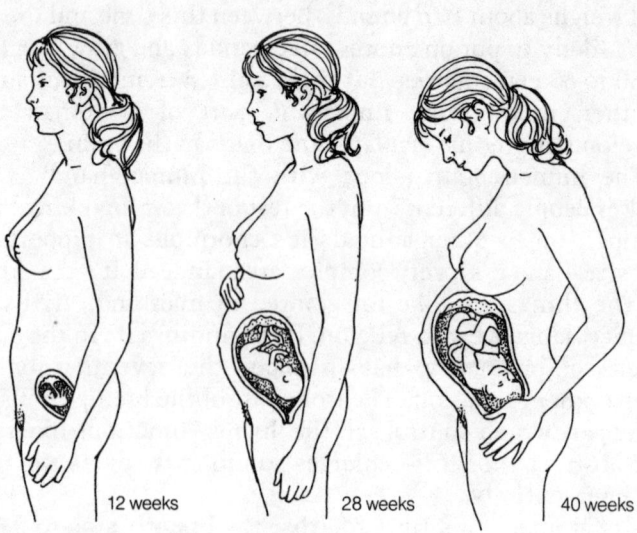

YOUR CHANGING SHAPE

12 weeks   28 weeks   40 weeks

sleep – short for *rapid eye movement*. Using special machines to monitor babies in the womb, researchers have discovered that they exhibit the same sorts of brain waves, so even if we can't see their eyes moving, it's almost certain that something is going on in their brains. Even more interestingly, it's been found that very often mothers and their babies in the womb exhibit 'dreaming' brain patterns at the same time – that is, they're probably dreaming together.

What does a baby in the womb dream about? Nobody knows, though oddly enough, it's something we all did once. Some scientists have gone so far as to speculate that there might even be some sort of telepathic link between a mother and her baby in the womb, a link which operates when the two 'dream together'. This 'dream bridge', they say, might explain why some children seem to have 'memories' of things which happened before they were born. Perhaps while mother and baby dream, fragments of consciousness pass from one to the other.

Of course, something like this is very hard to prove but I still find it a powerful symbol of how close mother and baby are during pregnancy.

5. Being Pregnant

LET'S START with the most obvious changes pregnancy brings about; those in a woman's body. It's important to remember that all the changes have a very definite purpose, and that's to make sure the body can carry the baby through pregnancy, give birth and provide food for her afterwards in the form of breast milk. There are also side effects of the processes which make these things possible.

The processes themselves are controlled by the hormones *oestrogen* and *progesterone*. These hormones suppress ovulation, and also stimulate the milk glands in the breasts to begin developing, something which can make the breasts very tender in the early months of pregnancy.

Of course, the most visible change is the growth of a pregnant woman's abdomen. This is caused by the baby growing in the womb, which is a quite remarkable organ. It is one large muscle, and the fibres out of which it's made are capable of stretching up to forty times their original length – which they do, as the baby grows. The growth of the womb means other organs inside the body are pushed out of the way, something which, amazingly enough, has very little effect on them. One problem it does cause quite often is an increased need to urinate – the result of simple, physical pressure from the womb on the nearby bladder.

Women usually gain weight fairly steadily throughout pregnancy, and other areas where they might put on some extra inches are around the hips, thighs and buttocks and the breasts. I'll have more to say about weight gain a little further on, but it's enough to say here that the extra weight coupled with the demands the baby makes on the mother's system mean that pregnant women's bodies have to work harder to do the things they've always done – such as walking, carrying bags, climbing stairs and so on. In fact, during pregnancy, a woman's heart works up to 40 per cent harder. That's also partly because she has more blood in her system to help supply the baby's needs – between 25 and 40 per cent more, in all. Linked to this is the fact that she even breathes in more air for the baby. Before pregnancy, each breath takes in about 500 cubic centimetres of air; during pregnancy it's more like 800 cubic centimetres.

Doctors think it is the fluctuating levels of hormones in a woman's system which causes one of the best known early signs of pregnancy – *nausea*. Many people think that this always appears in the form of morning sickness and involves lots of vomiting. The truth is that it needn't happen in the morning, and it also needn't mean actual vomiting. Some women *are* sick, but many just feel nauseous, sometimes in the morning, sometimes in the evening – and some unlucky women feel sick all day.

Doctors also think that hormones – linked with the other changes of pregnancy – are the cause of another symptom, *tiredness*. Some women do become extremely tired in the early months of pregnancy, even to the extent that they can't carry on a normal life. Again, this varies from woman to woman, but many find that they're much more tired than usual, even if they actually do less!

Some mothers also notice early on in pregnancy – especially women with dark complexions – that their skins change colour slightly in certain areas. The most usual places to be affected are the nipples and the *areolae* (the area surrounding the nipple), and the tendency is for them to become darker. Others also develop a dark line running down the stomach from navel to pubic hair – it's called the *linea negra*, which is simply the Latin for 'black line'. Others find they have darker patches of skin on their faces over the cheeks and forehead. It sometimes looks like a butterfly, and that's why it's called a *butterfly mask*. Moles and birthmarks may also become darker. All these changes are side effects of the raised levels of hormones in the system, and none of them are permanent. After the birth, your skin is almost certain to return to its former state.

Being uncomfortable

You may have come to realise by now that pregnancy can be quite an uncomfortable condition. Most of the women I know would agree with that statement, anyway – and some would say that it can be very uncomfortable indeed. Nausea and tiredness can make the first three months of pregnancy very unpleasant, and some women suffer from them throughout the nine months. But there are other problems too, most of which come under the heading of side effects.

For example, as a pregnant woman's abdomen grows, there's going to be an increasing strain on her back. This problem is made worse because those hormones in the system also tend to make ligaments and muscles all over the body softer and looser than normal. That means they can't stand as much strain as usual before aching – all of which adds up to backache for pregnant women, and few manage to avoid it.

Those ever-present hormones also tend to slow down the movement of the bowel, and generally make it more sluggish than usual. This can lead to constipation, which can be made worse by a poor diet lacking in fibre. In some cases the straining constipation causes can lead to the appearance of swollen, painful veins in the anus, a condition known as *piles* (haemorrhoids). Again, the hormones may add fuel to the fire (so to speak) because they also tend to make the veins in that area softer and looser than usual anyway.

Some pregnant women also suffer from more wind or gas than usual, another result of pressure on the other organs from the womb. Heartburn is another common problem, as are odd skin rashes (probably caused by sweating in folds of skin under the enlarged abdomen or breasts) and cramp. You have a higher chance of getting *thrush* during pregnancy, too. This is a fungal infection of the vagina which can be dealt with easily by fungicides – but it's often quite painful. In later pregnancy the sheer size of a woman's abdomen may make life very difficult. She'll certainly feel tired, and she may even begin to feel a little breathless – the result of all the extra work her body has to do, plus the cramping effect on her lungs of the growing womb.

She'll also find it hard to do things like cut her toe nails – she won't be able to bend over.

And there are, of course, two other problems which many young women worry about when they become pregnant – *stretch marks* and *varicose veins*. These last – unsightly, swollen veins in the legs – are caused by damaged valves in the deep leg veins which make the blood collect in 'pools'. It is therefore harder for it to get back to the heart. As with piles, the extra hormones of pregnancy play a part in this; there's an added strain on the veins because of the increased amount of progesterone in the blood which makes them more relaxed. Not taking enough exercise and standing too long can also be contributory factors.

Stretch marks are a different matter, though. These are exactly what they sound like, marks in the skin caused by stretching. They usually appear as pink or red lines round areas where weight is put on, such as the breasts, abdomen, thighs or buttocks, although obviously which areas are affected and how much varies greatly from woman to woman. After the birth, when the skin begins to go back to normal, the stretch marks turn silvery white. The bad news is that they're permanent. Once they've happened, they stay for life.

Doctors were mystified by stretch marks until quite recently, and had no idea what caused them. It seemed to have very little to do with how much weight a woman put on, for example. Some women who put on large amounts of weight in pregnancy didn't get them while other women who put on very little did – or vice versa. There was no way of telling beforehand whether you'd get them or not, and nothing you could do afterwards.

It's now thought, however, that a tendency to have stretch marks could be inherited – and also that it's got a lot to do with the sort of food you eat (or rather don't eat) during your adolescence. Stretch marks are actually tears in the layers underneath the surface of the skin caused by expansion. When the skin goes back to normal, the tears remain as scars. Doctors now know that it's important to get plenty of a mineral called *zinc* during the crucial growing periods of your teenage years to make these layers under the skin as supple as possible. If you didn't get enough, it means they'll tear under less pressure than in someone who did – and you'll have stretch marks. Doctors still can't do anything about them once they've appeared, but if you want to do your best to avoid them, it's sensible to eat the sort of diet I described in Chapter 3 – which will be more than likely to give you enough zinc.

Love it or loathe it?

With all this going on, it's not surprising that some women should dislike pregnancy, or at least, large parts of it. In fact some women – and I've talked to a few who feel this way – loathe the whole experience from start to finish.

Of course, how much *you* enjoy anything in life depends on many things, and pregnancy is no exception. It will, of course, depend on your personality, how much you suffer from the problems I've talked about in this chapter, how much you wanted to have a baby in the first place, your personal circumstances, your relationship, and so on. Of course, it's also important to remember that your feelings might change during the period of pregnancy, and also that different women feel different about it.

How much you enjoy pregnancy also depends to a large extent on your *perception* of the experience. Many women I've talked to said that their main worry about becoming pregnant was that it would ruin their bodies for the rest of their lives. "Being pregnant just made me feel fat and ugly," said one woman. "I felt completely unattractive." This is a very common experience; most pregnant women find their changed shape unattractive, some much more than others.

But why should this be so? Why should a woman who is pregnant think she is ugly all of a sudden? After all, pregnancy is a completely normal, natural event. It's associated with the good things in life, like love, children, the continuation of the human race. It can involve discomfort and some problems – but why should it be thought of as something ugly?

Society, however, decrees certain standards of feminine beauty. Girls are taught from a very early age that to be beautiful you have to be slim and slender, perhaps even thin.

Of course they might not be taught this directly; but the assumption that beauty and being slim go hand in hand is all around us, on the television, in newspapers, magazines, commercials and so on.

It's important to realise that this hasn't always been so. In the Middle Ages, for example, pregnancy was often considered to be the most beautiful female condition of all. Fashions – like high-waisted dresses which emphasised the abdomen – were designed to make even non-pregnant women look as if they were expecting a baby. Today's fashions do the opposite. Tight jeans are designed to emphasise – perhaps even exaggerate – the narrow waist which pregnancy soon obliterates. And many maternity clothes seem to have been made to *conceal* the fact that a woman is pregnant rather than to flaunt it. In essence, today's ideal woman is the slim model or dancer; and certainly not the Madonna and child of the Middle Ages.

All this affects your perception of pregnancy. Even if you really want a baby and start off feeling very positive, with this sort of social background you'll probably find yourself having at least a few second thoughts, especially in the early months. Part of this is the sudden shock we all experience when something we've wanted for a long time becomes a reality. There's no doubt that the moment when a pregnancy is confirmed is just like that. "Suddenly it was definite, confirmed," one woman said to me. "I was really surprised, even though we'd been trying for a baby. It seemed unreal. From that moment, everything seemed to take on a momentum of its own, and we were swept along."

Friends and relatives begin to congratulate you and say things like "You must be so pleased", when you might be starting to wonder what on earth you've got yourself into. It's vital that you should remember one thing above all at this time – it's perfectly normal to feel this way, and most first time parents do, even if they claim they don't. However little you know about what's coming – and those of you who read this book will know a lot more – you still know that pregnancy, childbirth and becoming a parent represents a major change in your life. If you didn't feel a little confused, nervous, even anxious about it at all, then you'd be a very odd human being indeed. Add to this the fact that you might be suffering from nausea and fatigue and you'll begin to see why early pregnancy can be a time when your feelings are less than positive. In fact you can feel *very* miserable if you're one of the few women who suffer seriously from both those two problems.

Middle and later pregnancy can have their troubles, too. There are the purely physical problems, but there can be others, too, like people's attitudes: "All of a sudden," one woman said, "*I* wasn't *me* any more. People started talking to the baby in my womb rather than me. It seemed that I'd become a mum, and that meant I'd stopped being a person in my own right."

I talked about anxiety above, and anxiety and fear are closely related emotions. No description of people's feelings about pregnancy would be complete without mentioning fear. Most women – in fact all the ones I've talked to, and more than a few of their partners as well – have one main fear which can sometimes be almost overwhelming. It's the fear that there might be something wrong with that child inside the womb, that she might be handicapped in some way.

Some women have very strange dreams during their pregnancies, even nightmares, often involving these sorts of fears. Both Sally and I worried that we wouldn't be able to love our babies enough, and it's important to remember that this sort of uncertainty is very common. Some women feel guilty because of these secret thoughts and fears, but there's absolutely no need to.

Another very common fear – and one which few women will admit to – is fear of birth itself. Almost all women spend at least some of their pregnancies wondering how painful birth is going to be, and whether they're going to be able to cope with it. Obviously, some women worry more about this than others, and something which is very clear is that the more you know about birth, the less likely you are to be afraid of it. And various studies have shown that if this is the case, then you're likely to have an easier birth.

It has to be said, though, that there are women who love the experience of pregnancy. For women who have few problems and who are relaxed and confident, being pregnant can actually make them feel happier, healthier and more at peace. There's also the legendary 'pregnancy bloom' which some women get, and I know there are many men – I'm one of them – who say that their wives can look stunning while they're expecting a baby. The middle part of pregnancy can be especially peaceful and happy; that's the time when any nausea and fatigue is likely to have lessened in effect at the very least, and maybe even have disappeared, and the 'bump' still isn't so big that it makes life uncomfortable. One woman I know said to me it was at this stage that she felt as if she didn't want her pregnancy to end: "I wanted it just to go on for ever and ever."

And there are other women, with even more reason for loving the experience of being pregnant, even if the pregnancy is riddled with problems and very difficult. It's very much a question of perception. I know one woman who tried to get pregnant for several years before she finally achieved it, and was very worried for a time that she would never have a baby at all. She then had to put up with severe nausea throughout her pregnancy, as well as several other more serious health problems.

"Quite frankly I didn't care," she told me. "I was so desperate to have a baby that if they'd said I'd have to have my leg cut off to do so, I wouldn't have blinked. And even though I felt dreadful all through my pregnancy, I'd still say I loved being pregnant. It meant so much to me to know that *my* baby was on the way."

Going to the doctor

Of course the first thing you should do if you think you're pregnant is go to your doctor. He'll be able to confirm whether you are or not by arranging a simple test. You'll be asked for a sample of urine. This is tested chemically in a laboratory for the presence of pregnancy hormones. There are some very reliable and inexpensive do-it-yourself pregnancy testing kits on the market these days as well, and they make finding out whether you are pregnant very easy indeed.

It's important to have a pregnancy confirmed as early as possible for several reasons. The first is that the earlier you know you're pregnant, the more time you've got to do something about it if you're unhappy with the idea or there's some other reason you might need to have an abortion.

If you decide to continue with the pregnancy, it is important to remember that the baby is very vulnerable during the first three months in the womb. You need to avoid certain things to make sure your baby has the best possible chance of developing normally. For example, X-rays should be avoided wherever possible, even though the risk is quite small in most cases. Doctors these days advise women only to have X-rays – even dental ones – in the fortnight just *after* they've had a period so they can be absolutely certain they're not pregnant.

Your doctor will also probably take steps at this first appointment to start making arrangements for your *antenatal care*. This simply means 'care before the birth', and it's probably the most important thing which happens to you throughout your pregnancy. How it's handled varies from country to country, and even from area to area inside countries. But wherever you live, it's likely that when you become pregnant your doctor will arrange for you to have regular check-ups. The point of these check-ups is simple. By keeping an eye on you during your pregnancy, your doctor can detect any problems early on. This will give him plenty of time to take the right action – and that could mean the difference between saving your baby's life or not.

In the United Kingdom, many women see their family doctors for antenatal care for most of their pregnancy, and in the later weeks, a doctor at the hospital where they're going to give birth. They'll also see a *midwife* regularly; she's a nurse who has had a long additional training so that she is able to handle normal antenatal care and childbirth. I say *she* because the vast majority of midwives are women – several men have become qualified midwives in Britain in recent years, but they're very, very few and far between.

You'll probably see a doctor or midwife every four weeks or so up to 28 weeks of pregnancy, then every two weeks up to about 36 weeks, and then every week after that. At your first antenatal appointment – it's usually called your *booking-in appointment* – you'll be asked all sorts of questions about your medical history. This isn't just being nosy on the part of your doctor – it's so he can work out whether there's anything about you which makes pregnancy particularly risky in your case. You'll be asked for a blood sample, and this will be tested for several things. First, it's tested to see if you've got any diseases which might cause problems. It's also tested to see if you're *anaemic* – that is, whether you've got enough iron in your system – and also to make sure you're immune to German measles. You'll also be given a full examination and weighed, your blood pressure will be taken, and you'll be asked to provide a urine sample for analysis. If you're anaemic you may be given iron tablets, and advised to eat more *folic acid*, which is found in green vegetables.

Remember that the reason you have regular check-ups is so that your doctor can build up a picture of how your pregnancy is going. That's why subsequent visits will be fairly similar to that first one. Your blood pressure and weight will be checked again, and you'll be asked for more urine samples, for example. As your abdomen grows, he'll also begin to *palpate* it – this is a special way of feeling it with his hands to check on the size of the womb and the baby's position in it. He may also listen for the baby's heartbeat through an ear trumpet, which he presses against your abdomen.

There are some other, more sophisticated tests which can also be done these days. One of the most common is called *ultrasound*. In this, a special machine is used to pass sound waves through the womb. The harmless echoes 'bounce' off the baby, and the resulting signals are fed into a television screen, producing a 'picture' of the baby in the womb. It checks that the baby is developing normally, and in some hospitals it's offered to all pregnant women.

Another test is called an *amniocentesis*. This involves inserting a fine needle into the womb and drawing off some of the amniotic fluid which surrounds the baby – hence the name. This fluid can tell doctors many things about the baby, including whether she's physically handicapped in certain ways. It's used to check on exactly that; once a couple know their child is handicapped, they can then opt for an abortion if they wish. However, it takes a long time for the results of the test to be known, and abortions after amniocentesis are usually quite late – and therefore sometimes distressing.

On the conveyor belt

It is vital to keep all your antenatal appointments, although it can seem a waste of time if all your doctor or midwife say when you go is "Fine, nothing to worry about." It can seem even more of a waste of time if you aren't treated the right way and, unfortunately, that can happen too.

"I just felt as if I was on a conveyor belt," said one woman. "I was being swept along, poked, prodded, examined, discussed. They took my blood and my urine, and didn't answer my questions. They made me feel as if *I* didn't matter. It was all so impersonal."

One of the biggest problems of modern life is that medicine – especially in large hospitals – can be very impersonal. In recent years many women, stimulated by the movement to gain more freedom for their sex in all areas of life, have heavily criticised antenatal care in particular. It is a fact that women often face long waits in antenatal clinics, that they're seen by different doctors and midwives each time they have an appointment, that their questions and concerns aren't answered or dealt with. But it seems that under the barrage of criticism things – at least in Britain – are beginning to change, and that antenatal care is developing a more human face.

However, it's important for you to remember that if you're unhappy with the sort of antenatal care you're getting, it's up to you to speak up and to do something about it. Doctors and midwives are human, so they can't be expected to be nice all the time; even saints must have their off days. But if you feel like a slab of meat on a conveyor belt, that's not going to make it easy for you to enjoy your pregnancy. It's your body and your baby, and the better you feel about the care you're getting, the easier life will be for you. Take a list of the questions you want to ask so you don't forget. Ask for anything you don't understand to be explained, and don't stop asking until you've got an answer which satisfies you. It can be very difficult to have the courage to do this; we tend to treat doctors and other medical unhappy.

Preparing for birth

One thing that good antenatal care will do is to give you a chance to talk things over with someone who knows about what you're going through. Not all doctors or midwives are good at this, but many are. They'll give you a chance to talk about your feelings, ask questions and help you to overcome the secret fears and anxieties which can make pregnancy an unsettling time.

One thing your doctor or midwife will do very early on is suggest you go to some *antenatal classes*. Most maternity hospitals run these, although there are some organisations which run them privately, like the National Childbirth Trust in Britain (see page 188). The main emphasis in these classes is on learning how to get through labour. You'll probably be taught all about birth and how you're likely to feel during it. You'll also be taught relaxation and breathing exercises to help you cope with the pain of giving birth.

But what you learn at these classes doesn't end there. You'll be given some basic information on how to care for your baby, for example. This will range from how to breastfeed or bottle feed successfully, to how to change your baby's nappy or give her a bath. If you're lucky, your class teacher – who's likely to be a midwife – will arrange for a new mother to come along with a real live baby and demonstrate how these things are done.

Antenatal classes are valuable for more than all this, though. They also give you a chance to meet other people who are in the same boat as you. "I thought I was the only pregnant woman ever to feel so ignorant or nervous," one woman told me. "Then I went to antenatal classes and was delighted to find that everyone felt the same way." You may make friends who'll be a great help to you in the difficult months of early parenthood, and friends can be very important at such a time.

A positive approach

Making the decision to go to antenatal classes can be daunting, especially if you're shy. But it's an important, *positive* thing to do – and that word is the key to making your experience of pregnancy an enjoyable one.

All those things I talked about earlier – the insomnia, the sickness and the cramps – they're all things which happen *to* you. It often seems to pregnant women that they have no control over their lives – and particularly their bodies – any more. In this sense, being pregnant can come to feel like a very *passive* state.

But there are many positive things you can do which will help you to avoid all those problems. No one can guarantee that if you follow a certain régime you'll have no discomfort or problems at all. But you can minimise the problems without too much effort. This is where we come back to the guidelines for healthy living I've been talking about ever since Chapter 3.

Doctors vary in their estimates of how much weight you should put on in pregnancy, but they all agree on one thing. It's vital not to put on too much. There are a couple of other points to consider, too. Although I've said that stretch marks are sometimes unavoidable, the less weight you put on, the less your skin will have to stretch – and the less you'll be marked if they happen to you. And don't forget that the more weight you put on, the harder it will be to get your figure back once the baby is born.

Most doctors say that a weight gain of between 20 and 28 pounds by the end of pregnancy is about right. It might sound a lot if you consider that an average baby weighs about seven and a half pounds at birth. But the placenta will weigh over a pound, and the fluid in the womb is likely to weigh up to two pounds. The womb itself has got much bigger – and therefore heavier – and so have the breasts. And all that extra blood in the system probably adds another four pounds or so. But that still leaves a good few pounds of simple fat.

How much *you* will put on depends on several factors. It depends on your size and build, as well as the sort – and amount — of food you eat. Obviously, bigger women, especially if their partners are big as well, will tend to have bigger babies, and therefore put on more weight, although it might all be in proportion; the reverse is also true, with smaller women tending to have smaller babies, and so on.

But taking positive steps to make sure your diet is right both for you and your growing baby will be one of the best things you can do. Being positive about exercise will help, too. Nobody's suggesting that you take up gymnastics or marathon running during your pregnancy; there's a very good case for being careful not to over-exert yourself, and it's wise to take your doctor's advice about any strenuous activity you intend to take up while you're pregnant. But there are plenty of activities around which will give you some exercise in a gentler, but just as valuable way. Many pregnant women are taking up yoga, and there are courses run specifically to help women in pregnancy and childbirth. Walking, swimming, cycling — all these things can help you to feel fitter, healthier and happier.

Many women also keep their spirits up in pregnancy by making sure they look after their bodies from a beauty point of view. Pregnancy can affect your skin, and some women also have a few problems with their hair. Giving skin and hair extra care, perhaps even treating yourself to things you've never had before like a manicure, or an expensive new hairstyle, if you can afford it, may make you feel a lot happier. Good skin care can also help you to avoid any rashes.

It's also important to take a positive approach to looking after your breasts during pregnancy so that you'll be able to breastfeed your baby. I said that the development of the milk glands in the breasts may actually make them feel quite tender during the early months. They'll probably stay tender — although a little less so — throughout the nine months. Most doctors say that it's important to wear a good supporting bra from early on.

At around five months, many women find that their breasts produce a clear, yellow fluid. This is called *colostrum*, and it's the first food your baby will get from the breast. If it's left, colostrum can form crusts on the nipples which will make them sore. So you need to wash your breasts regularly, making sure that no crusts form. I believe that breastfeeding is the best way to feed your baby, and that's what the experts think, too. Not everyone finds it easy, though, and you'll be doing yourself – and your baby – a favour if you take positive steps during pregnancy to make sure you can do it successfully. Many women, for example, massage oil into their nipples to keep them supple in readiness for feeding, and even learn to express their milk by hand. This means squeezing the breast so that milk flows – a technique which will come in very handy later on.

Your relationship

A positive approach will also pay off in your relationship, which can begin to show signs of strain early on in pregnancy. I haven't said much specifically about men so far; but the sort of problems men face in their partners' pregnancies will throw light on how a relationship fares during this testing time.

Something very few men realise is that they too can suffer from physical symptoms in their partners' pregnancies. In 1965, two British psychiatrists carried out some research on prospective fathers. They discovered that many of them suffered from a whole range of physical symptoms during pregnancy, some of which affected them quite seriously.

These symptons included things like loss of appetite, nausea and even vomiting – symptoms very similar to those their wives might have been suffering at the same time. They also suffered from indigestion, stomach pains, constipation and diarrhoea. There were other, more vague and general problems that they complained of, too: headaches, bad nerves, general weakness, fatigue, depression, irritability, insomnia – and even food cravings. They didn't discover anyone who'd actually had a 'sympathetic pregnancy', so this particular myth, the one where a husband's abdomen swells like his wife's during pregnancy, is probably just that, a myth, and nothing more. But a few husbands were actually found to be suffering just as much – some even a little more – than their wives.

This sort of male reaction to pregnancy is very common. I know I had many of those symptoms during all three of Sally's pregnancies. I hope this doesn't sound too egotistical, but I think my experience is a perfect example, and explains why men react in this way.

It wasn't all that long ago that doctors began to confirm something most people have known for thousands of years; that is, if someone you love is going through something difficult, and especially if that person is suffering or in pain, then *you* may end up suffering in very much the same way simply out of empathy. When two people love each other and live together, they may reach the stage where anything that one goes through will affect the other. I know that I felt very upset about Sally's nausea and extreme tiredness in her pregnancies, and worried that things might not be going right.

The mention of worry brings me to the other reason why I didn't feel too good. And that's *stress*. Pregnancy is a time of anxiety and stress for most men, just as it is for their partners. In fact, those symptoms I listed above are the classic, physical signs of too much stress in anyone, let alone a 'pregnant father'. Men are under stress in this situation because the imminent arrival of their child represents just as big a change in their lives as it does for their partners.

Girls are brought up – even though their parents might do it unconsciously – to think of themselves as 'potential mothers'. Even if they eventually discover that babies aren't for them, this sort of pressure and these assumptions at least give girls *some* sort of preparation for parenthood.

Boys don't even get that. Girls get the dolls, boys get the guns. Boys are encouraged to be tough, outgoing, sporty, independent – and they're also not supposed to show their feelings; big boys don't cry, after all. Of course, the problem is that most boys do end up being fathers; and none of their upbringing has prepared them for the shock of becoming a parent at all. In a sense, coping with parenthood is, for many men, very difficult indeed; perhaps even more difficult in the initial stages than for their partners.

Two things tend to happen to men during pregnancy. The first is that they suddenly feel incredibly *responsible*, even burdened with responsibility. Their carefree, bachelor days are finally over; now they are about to become family men, fathers with a *duty* to support their families. Even men whose partners intend to work while their children are very small have told me that they still feel this way. For men whose partners are going to give up work – however temporarily – money and providing a secure environment for this new family of three people suddenly can become a major source of anxiety.

The second thing to happen to many men is that they begin to feel isolated, left out. Many men feel that their partners are getting all the limelight; they're the ones on whom all the attention is focussed. It's true that pregnant fathers do tend to be ignored, and there's even a lot of resistance to the idea that men should 'suffer' or have feelings in pregnancy at all. We're expected to put a brave face on it and slip into the background. So you find yourself in a very difficult position. There you are, worrying about your partner's nausea and fatigue, anxious about how you're going to cope financially, worried that you won't make a very good parent, and generally discovering that you're swimming in deep – and for you – uncharted waters. And nobody is taking any notice.

Except, perhaps, your partner. The important thing to remember here is that a baby can come between a couple, however much they love each other. It can start in pregnancy. A man might feel that his partner isn't taking any notice of his feelings; she might seem totally wrapped up in herself and the baby she's carrying. Inevitably, he becomes jealous of that baby before she's even born, and unhappy with his partner. It's a recipe for trouble which has soured many marriages. It can also happen the other way around; if a man seems to be wrapped up in the idea of the baby, his partner may well begin to feel that she doesn't matter to him as a person, and become just as jealous or unhappy.

It's something I've seen, and, like most couples, even experienced myself – a little. It's very easy, as we'll see, for a couple to split into two separate halves and begin to live in totally separate worlds. Men who are unsure of their abilities as parents and frightened of the whole process of becoming a parent because they're unprepared for it, often retreat into work or their hobbies, and leave it all to their partners. The latter then feel deserted, isolated; they need help and don't get it. Arguments blow up, and under the enormous pressure of being the parents of a small baby, many young couples find themselves deeply unhappy.

The point I always try to keep in mind is that you're in it *together*. Nobody can cope with parenthood completely alone all the time; and nobody will get the best out of parenthood without some relief and help. There's a point to be made here about men, too; more and more men – like myself – are coming to realise that being the traditional 'breadwinner' who leaves child care to his partner means he misses out on a lot. I enjoy my children; I want to share as much of their childhood with Sally as I can. The way to make sure you can do this is to share everything – as far as possible – right from the beginning.

In very simple terms, it seems that couples who talk together about their feelings generally get on better in pregnancy and afterwards. If you both understand a little of what you're each going through – and show some sympathy – then you're off to a flying start. Men can go along to their partners' relaxation and antenatal classes – there's often a 'fathers' night' – and try to find out as much as they can about birth and having children. Most fathers these days also choose to be at the births of their children, and that's probably the most important thing a man can do at the beginning of his transition to parenthood. Remember – stress is an integral part of that process, and we all cope better with stress if we've got support. Who better to give it to – and to receive it from – than the person you love, your 'co-parent'?

Enjoying pregnancy

You might be thinking by now that it's impossible to enjoy pregnancy as a couple; it sounds as if there's far too much to worry about. But many couples *do* enjoy it, and for them it's a time of great closeness and togetherness. Various research studies have thrown up some interesting facts about this. For example, couples who have a positive experience of pregnancy tend to cope better with the shocks of the early months of parenthood. It's also been shown that men who take an interest in their partners' pregnancies are often also more interested and involved with their partners and children *after* the birth, which makes life pleasanter and easier for everybody – mother, father and baby.

There are lots of things about pregnancy which couples enjoy. First and foremost, particularly for those couples who have made a conscious decision to have a child, there's the thrill of watching this amazing physical process unfold. I'll never forget feeling my first child kick inside her mother's abdomen; it's a feeling which has to be experienced to be believed, and it's one which loses none of its magic in subsequent pregnancies.

There are the funny things, too; when Sally was eight months pregnant she discovered that she couldn't bend in the middle enough to cut her own toe nails, so I had to do it for her. That was certainly something which neither of us had foreseen as being part of parenthood! There's the fun – and the arguments – you have choosing names for your child. You'll probably find that each name which is suggested conjures up visions of people you either don't like or don't want your child to resemble. And like most people, you'll probably reject the names of your partner's former girlfriends or boyfriends – and with good reason, too!

Your parents are also bound to join in the fun – and embarrass you endlessly – by telling stories about you and your brothers and sisters, uncles, aunts, cousins and friends as children and babies. The imminent arrival of a new member of the family can stir everyone's memories. It can get on your nerves, sometimes; but it's often a source of pleasure, a confirmation of belonging to a wider circle of family.

But despite all this, many young couples worry about one of the things which can serve to draw them closely together during pregnancy – their sexual relationship. There are a lot of old wives' tales about sex in pregnancy, and a strong sense in many people that it's wrong in some way. Many men worry a lot that sex will harm the baby – but they couldn't be more wrong.

In general, doctors say that couples can continue their sex lives throughout pregnancy. Women who are in danger of having a miscarriage (a subject we'll be looking at in the next section) will be advised to be careful about sex, and to avoid it for a while if there's still a risk of losing the baby. And of course, many women find that the sickness and nausea of early pregnancy put them off sex, and in late pregnancy, the sheer size of a woman's abdomen can mean lovemaking becomes a little uncomfortable, to say the least.

Sex in pregnancy, however, can be a much more relaxed, stress-free pleasure than it was before. Many couples find that not having to worry about contraception means that sex is a lot less worrying. If this makes a couple happier, then it's not only good for them, it's good for the baby they're expecting. If she can come into a family in which her mother and father are close, she can't hope for a better start. Physical closeness is a good basis for emotional closeness – and that's something any young, new family needs as it sets out to face the stresses and strains of parenthood.

When things go wrong

Most women find that their pregnancies go smoothly from start to finish without any major problems. This wasn't always the case; in the past, various complications of pregnancy which we now consider to be minor even resulted in the death of mother or child, or both.

The main difference is that nowadays antenatal check-ups mean that almost all the most serious problems are picked up early enough to be treated with some measure of success. Doctors now have an enormous range of techniques to help them make sure pregnancy and birth have a successful outcome – the birth of a healthy child to a healthy mother. These techniques range from drugs to slow down a premature labour, to surgery for emergencies.

The routine tests at your antenatal check-ups are designed to detect certain specific problems. For example, your blood pressure will be taken regularly because if it's consistently high, it can put a strain on your heart and blood vessels, which are working over-time in pregnancy anyway. It can also harm your baby if it stays too high for too long, making it difficult for the placenta to work properly. Rest and relaxation is the usual treatment for this sort of high blood pressure.

It can also be the first sign of a dangerous illness called *pre-eclampsia*, though. In this, the high blood pressure, if undetected, can lead to the mother having a fit and the baby suffering seriously – or even dying – through lack of oxygen. Other signs of this illness are swelling, particularly of the hands and feet, and protein in the urine – which is why urine samples are taken at your antenatal check-ups. Pre-eclampsia is usually spotted early on; women who are found to be suffering from it are admitted to hospital for complete bed rest.

Some pregnancies do end in a *miscarriage*. Indeed, it's now thought that many pregnancies – especially first pregnancies – end very early, before a woman even suspects she's pregnant in most cases. What she thinks is just a slightly heavier period than usual is actually an unsuccessful embryo being cleared out of the womb. Doctors now think that these early miscarriages – and some even say that as many as one in ten pregnancies end in this way – are nature's way of correcting a mistake. For many of these miscarried embryos have been found to be abnormal in some way; that means that if the pregnancy had continued, the result would have been the birth of a handicapped baby.

In very many cases, however, doctors can never be sure exactly what it is that causes any particular miscarriage. They divide them into two categories, depending on when they happen. *Early miscarriages* much the most common, are those which occur before the thirteenth week of pregnancy; *late miscarriages* are those which happen after that. The latter shade into premature labour where the baby doesn't survive because she's too immature.

Very often, the first sign of a threatened miscarriage is some bleeding, and perhaps a little pain, possibly in the lower back. If it happens, your doctor will advise you to take to your bed immediately. So long as the cervix stays closed, there's every chance that the pregnancy will continue. If it's open, then there's no hope. Doctors also have drugs these days which they can use to try and slow down or stop a premature labour in later pregnancy.

Often it's a weak cervix which causes late miscarriages. The weakness means that the pregnancy is unstable, and women with this problem often have repeated miscarriages until it's sorted out. It's solved these days by actually stitching up the cervix to hold the pregnancy in. This technique is called a *Shirodkar stitch*; it's named after the doctor who invented it. The stitch is removed just before birth to allow the cervix to open in the normal way.

Miscarriage is a subject few people ever give any thought to until it happens to them. But a woman who has a miscarriage can feel very depressed about it for quite a while afterwards, sometimes even months. It's hard to believe unless you've got some experience of it, but you do actually grieve for the baby you have lost, even if the miscarriage is very early. It's something Sally and I have experience of; before she became pregnant with Thomas, our third child, she lost a baby at a couple of months. Both she and I felt very disturbed about it, and it was made worse because people seemed to expect us not to be upset about a miscarriage which happened so early. But you do feel that way – and you need to talk about it if you want to, you need sympathy, understanding, time. We both still wonder about that baby and what sort of child he or she might have been – and I think we always will.

6. Giving Birth

WHETHER YOU LOVE being pregnant or loathe it, you know one thing is certain at least – it has to come to an end. The inevitable end of your pregnancy is the birth of your child, and that end is, at the same time, the real beginning of your child's existence in the outside world.

Birth is an enormously important event for everyone concerned. That may sound a little obvious, but it's worth pausing at this stage just to think about it a little. Its importance for the baby is, of course, that it represents her first major step away from her parents and towards true independence. Until the moment of birth, she is dependent on her mother – in particular, the placenta and the umbilical cord – for *all* her needs. Birth is a physical separation, the moment when the baby has to take her first breath – or die. Anyone who's been present at such a moment will tell you that it's quite simply awe inspiring.

For the parents, it's the moment when they first meet the child they've been waiting for all through the nine months of pregnancy – and when they first meet themselves and each other in their new roles. Birth is the moment when they dive into the deep end of parenthood, and find out whether they're going to sink or swim. The circumstances of the birth itself – and how we perceive it – can play a vital role in determining what comes after.

Birth in three stages

Doctors divide the process by which a baby is born into three stages. And it's no accident that the name we give to this process – *labour* – should also mean *work*. There's no doubt about it; all the women I've talked to have said that labour is hard work, and the three labours I've been present at confirmed that as far as I was concerned. It looked like very hard work to me!

At any rate, labour is all about one organ in particular in a woman's body doing a lot of work. That organ is the womb, the baby's home throughout the nine months of her development. The *first stage of labour* is when the womb begins to contract in such a way that its neck (the cervix) opens up (or *dilates*) to a size large enough for the baby's head to pass through it. This can take some time, and the contractions come rhythmically, the gaps between them getting shorter and shorter until the cervix is open, and the womb and vagina form one unit with it – the *birth canal*. At that time, the cervix should be ten centimetres dilated.

The *second stage of labour* is when the baby is actually born – that is, when she passes from inside the womb to the outside world. This stage begins when the cervix is completely open and the mother feels she wants to push the baby out. In most births the head of the baby comes first, and this is the hardest part to push out. Once the widest part of the head is through the vaginal opening and can't slip back, it's said to have *crowned*. The rest of the baby's body usually comes fairly quickly and easily after that moment.

The *third stage of labour* is when the womb expels what's left inside after the baby's made her exit and entrance. Left behind is the placenta and umbilical cord (part of which will have come out with the baby). The placenta is called the *afterbirth*, for obvious reasons.

In those terms it probably all sounds very simple and straightforward. But, as you'll see, it can sometimes be very complicated. Nobody knows exactly how labour starts, for example. It probably has quite a lot to do with the baby and the fact that she grows to fill the womb; at any rate, we know that usually just before labour begins, the baby gives the placenta some sort of 'signal' – what it is we don't know – and the mother's pituitary gland then starts to produce lots of the hormone which stimulates the womb to contract.

Whatever the exact internal mechanism, doctors, midwives and women know what the first external signs of labour are. Many women have what's known as a 'show'. All through the pregnancy the cervix is blocked with a plug of thick mucus to keep the baby in and infection out. As the cervix begins to dilate this plug comes loose, and comes out of the vagina. Often it's stained with blood.

A large number of women also find that their 'waters break'. These waters are the amniotic fluid which surrounds the baby in the womb throughout pregnancy. In some women they burst dramatically and quite suddenly, flooding out of the vagina all at once. Others experience a slow seeping away over a period of time, while still others never notice it at all.

One thing above all characterises the onset of labour, and that's the pain of contractions. In fact the pregnant woman's womb 'practises' for the big day almost all the time. Most women can feel their wombs contracting during pregnancy, even quite early on. These 'trial contractions' – which doctors call *Braxton-Hicks contractions* – can become quite strong towards the end of pregnancy, and even lead you to suspect that you're going into labour before it really happens. Many women have these false alarms. They're usually nothing to worry about – and most women say that they're well aware of what's going on once the real thing starts!

In this connection it's important to remember that the womb of a woman who's never given birth before will take longer to do it than on any subsequent occasion. In a sense it's because the womb hasn't the experience. It's not surprising, therefore, that a first birth usually takes longer on average than second or later births. Figures vary, but the average length of labour – from the very beginning to the actual moment when the baby is born – is usually between twelve and fifteen hours for a first baby, six to nine hours for a second baby, less for a third and so on. One study I saw revealed that it takes about a 150 contractions to deliver a first baby, 75 for a second or third, 50 for a fourth or fifth.

At the beginning of labour a contraction might just feel like a twinge, and they're often first felt in the lower part of the back. This is because nerves from the pelvis – the area where all this is going on – at this point reach the spinal cord, along which they're transmitted to the brain. The pains might start off as much as twenty minutes apart and only last a few seconds; they take a while to build up steam.

But they do, rhythmically and unstoppably. Over a period of hours, they'll get stronger and stronger until they reach the stage where they seem to be coming all the time. By then you'll certainly be aware of them – and the pain that comes with them, too.

The pain of birth

Childbirth is something which happens every day. It's a natural, normal event – but it does involve pain. That's the one aspect of the experience which seems to worry most mothers beforehand. How will they cope with the pain?

One problem in this connection is that most of us grow up with some sort of idea of what birth is like. It's an idea we get from the stories we hear in our families, from books and magazines, from films and from television. Everyone's idea of birth is unique and reflects their own experiences, but as far as I can see there tend to be two ways of looking at it.

Imagine, if you will, two films, each featuring a birth. In the first, the heroine thrashes on a chaotic bed, screaming in agony, pouring with sweat, surrounded by midwives and doctors who call for hot water and clean sheets. The labour goes on for days, and our heroine expires soon after the baby appears. The heroine of our second film, however, does nothing so dramatic. She, in fact, is hardly seen; perhaps all we see is her husband pacing restlessly outside the room where she labours. Eventually he is ushered in to see his wife, who is lying in bed with her make-up perfect and not a hair out of place, cuddling a clean, quiet baby.

We've all seen films like that – and it doesn't take much imagination to realise that they're not exactly accurate in their portrayal of birth. In fact, most women I've talked to about it haven't got much patience with the way birth is portrayed in stories and on the screen. "It's just not true to life in most films," said one. "Birth hurts, there's no doubt about it. Anyone who goes into it expecting it to be painless is going to be very shocked indeed. But for most women it isn't all thrashing and screaming and agony either."

The first point to be made is that we all have different *pain thresholds* – that is, we all react to different amounts of pain in different ways. Some people pass out if they prick their thumbs with a pin, while others can cope with much higher levels of pain without even batting an eyelid. Nowhere is this more apparent than in birth. All the women I've talked to about it have different opinions. Some said it *was* agony, others that it didn't really hurt that much. Most said that it hurt but that they managed. How you cope with other sorts of pain doesn't seem to be much of a guideline to how you'll cope with birth, either; some women really surprised themselves.

Other things can affect your perception of pain in labour – like the attitude of the medical staff who attend you. But from the research that's been done, one thing seems clear above all; the more positive your approach to birth, the better your experience of it is likely to be.

A large part of this is mental preparation. The one advantage you have as far as the pains of birth are concerned is that you know you're going to have to experience them. So you can prepare to cope with them. That's why I recommended antenatal classes during pregnancy. That's where you'll be taught ways of doing exactly that, like breathing exercises, for example.

Anxiety and fear in pregnancy are often the results of not knowing what's going on. Imagine how much more afraid you're going to be if you don't know what's happening to you when you begin to give birth and the pains come. Any doctor will tell you, too, that pain is always worse when you're very frightened.

That's why it's important to know what's going on, to have prepared for birth. Then you'll know that the pains start off mild and get worse. You'll know that you can be helped by those around you, and that there are ways of coping. You'll know that however much it hurts, women throughout the ages have gone through it and survived to tell the tale. You'll also know that it's normal to be frightened – and also that you should try not to let the fear take over.

There's one very interesting theory about pain in birth. Some doctors have put forward the idea that the pain plays an important psychological role; by making birth difficult, they say, it makes women appreciate the result – the baby – all the more. I suppose there's an element of that in birth for many women; there's no doubt that they suffer to have their children. As a theory, though, it doesn't really hold water. The opposite could be true, with women rejecting the babies who cause them so much pain. Some women do actually reject their babies after birth – and who could blame a woman for feeling a little negative towards the cause of her pain? The theory also doesn't take into account that some lucky women do appear to have really pain-free births; some women have painkilling drugs or their babies delivered by Caesarean: and they all love their children just as much. One woman I know objected to this theory very strongly. "It must have been dreamed up by a man. You could only think that the pain makes you appreciate your baby more if you don't actually have to go through it!"

I thought that was a very fair point, and I must say that it feels unfair in some way for me – a man – to be talking about the pains of childbirth. But I have been present at three births, and I'm glad to say that Sally felt me being there made things a little easier for her, or so she said afterwards! That's something which research studies have backed up. These have shown that those women whose partners are with them during labour and birth have an easier time than those who labour alone – that is, without someone they know and love there to give them support. It's not hard to see why; having someone you trust and love with you at such a crucial time is bound to help. It's only right, after all, that both a child's parents should be there to greet her at birth – they were both present at her conception.

Like me, most modern fathers want to be present at the births of their children – and so they are. The figures vary, but it seems that something like eight or nine out of every ten fathers is in there with his partner helping her to get through birth. This is a relatively new development. It wasn't all that long ago – maybe even ten or fifteen years – that most men either stayed out of the delivery room on purpose or were kept out by the doctors and midwives. That's why you still see films and television programmes in which husbands pace up and down outside while their wives are delivering, even though it doesn't happen very often these days.

Some men genuinely can't face the idea, and it's not always because they're squeamish. I know that I found the sight of Sally in pain very upsetting, especially when I wasn't going through it – and I knew that I'd played a large part in causing it in the first place! If a man doesn't want to be there, it's up to him to discuss it with his partner. In the end, the only thing that matters is that the couple is really happy with the way their child is brought into the world. I will say one thing, though, to those males who don't like the idea; don't dismiss it out of hand. You might be surprised at just how much you enjoy the experience if you give it a try!

Before we move on to look at the other factors which can influence your experience of birth, I want to leave you with the words of one woman on the subject of pain. She is a friend, and someone I've interviewed about the births of her three children. She was especially positive about the last of her three births: "When Alice was born I felt that the pain was constructive. It was *clean* pain. I was in control and it was pain with a purpose."

Too much technology?

Unfortunately, many women have less than happy experiences of labour and birth. The problem seems to be a question of attitude on the part of doctors and medical staff. Many women I've talked to said that the most upsetting part of the whole process of becoming a parent was the feeling that doctors and midwives didn't really care about them as people. "Their attitude always seemed to be that they knew best and that I was so stupid I could safely be ignored."

The problem is widespread, and it isn't just restricted to pregnancy and birth. Our modern industrial society concentrates large numbers of people in cities, and in health terms this has led to the development of giant city hospitals. In these, doctors and midwives are very often rushed, and the system tends to turn everyone involved in it into people in a hurry, people who get irritated easily. First time mothers often seem to be the ones who lose out the most – the younger you are, the more frightening all this can seem, and the less certain you'll be. That might mean you'll be less assertive than you could be – and therefore less likely to get what you want. It's very easy to go along with someone who's considered to be an expert, someone like a doctor – even to the extent that you suppress any disagreements you might feel.

Many women get on very well with the medical staff who deliver their babies, most of whom are friendly, sympathetic and very helpful. No one in their sort of job can be an angel all the time, however, and it's important to remember this.

You can't really separate antenatal care and birth, and there have been many changes in recent years in attitudes towards ways of handling the delivery itself, again stimulated by the sort of criticism we've been talking about. Childbirth has become the centre of much heated debate.

On one side there are the people who say that there is far too much routine medical interference in birth; on the other side are those who point to the fact that it is the advances of modern medicine which have made childbirth as safe as it is today.

The first group says that for most women pregnancy and childbirth are perfectly natural processes with which the female body is designed to cope. Having a baby isn't an *illness*, after all, although few people would go as far as to say that problems never arise. Obviously, medicine – in the shape of experts who know how to deal with any problems that might crop up – has a major part to play.

The point is, say the critics, that childbirth has become so medicalised that for many women it isn't a natural event at all. By far the majority of women in most developed countries give birth in hospital, for example, and find themselves subjected to hospital routines. First time mothers may find themselves being *induced* before they know what's happening. This simply means bringing on labour artificially, and a variety of techniques are used to achieve it. Hormone pessaries are sometimes inserted into the vagina to stimulate the womb to contract. The same hormones can be fed into the bloodstream by an intravenous drip. The doctor may even break the membrane which holds the amniotic fluid in the womb to release it, something which should also get the contractions going. It's called *breaking the waters*. These techniques were devised to get babies out of the womb as quickly as possible if they were in any danger. Critics now say that they're used to suit the hospital's convenience, and that instead of waiting until a baby is born naturally, doctors sometimes use induction to fit births into *their* schedules. The problem is that the statistics show that induced labours are often longer and more painful than natural, spontaneous ones.

Other things about giving hospital birth can make the experience less than blissful. Hospitals have been known to have a policy of preparing women for birth. This meant shaving off the pubic hair and giving them an enema to empty their bowels, both things which campaigners say are unnecessary. Something else about which debate has raged is *episiotomy*. This is a cut in the vagina which a doctor or midwife makes at a crucial point in birth – usually just before the head is crowned – and which is supposed to make birth easier by enlarging the vagina at the right time. The skin in that area does sometimes tear under the pressure of birth. Some doctors claim that it's easier to repair an episiotomy than a tear – but critics point to the fact that many women have a lot of trouble with their stitches afterwards. In some hospitals almost three quarters of the mothers – and a higher proportion of first time mothers – have an episiotomy. Critics say that this can't be necessary.

It's also highly likely that a woman who gives birth in hospital will do so while lying on her back on a delivery couch. That might not sound like a problem, but there are some experts who have said that if there is such a thing as the worst possible position to give birth in, then it's lying on your back. Interestingly enough, it seems that in most societies and throughout history women have given birth in other – and more active – positions. There has been a lot of interest in recent years in so-called *active birth*, in which a woman is encouraged to move around as much as she wants to during labour and to take up the position for birth in which she feels most comfortable.

Supporters of this approach point to several facts. One is that women who give birth in this way, – some squat, some get on to their hands and knees – report less pain, have easier and shorter labours in general, and seem to enjoy it much more. Women who give birth lying on their backs seem to take longer, have more pain and need more help. The evidence also shows that babies of women who give birth in an active way seem to be happier and more lively from the start – which is understandable. Birth is quite a stressful event for the baby, too, and the less time and effort it takes, the better for her.

Another aspect of medicalised birth which has come in for criticism is the use of painkilling drugs. Various drugs are offered to women to help them cope with the pain; *gas and oxygen (Entonox)*, for example, which is breathed in through a mask during a contraction. There's also *pethidine*, a drug which is injected. There's an *epidural*, a technique in which anaesthetic is injected near a special part of the spine to numb the nerves carrying pain from the pelvis, and which should make the birth almost pain free.

The problems of drugs are quite simple. Pethidine, for example, can make a woman very drowsy, and passes across the placenta during birth to have the same effect on her baby. It may also make her feel less involved in the labour, or make the baby slow to start breathing. It can also affect the process of *bonding* after the birth. This is the technical term for the process by which mother and baby get to know each other, a process for which they both need to be fairly alert. Part of it involves getting breastfeeding established, and unless you get a good start with this, it's sometimes hard to keep it going later on. Epidurals, too, not only remove all pain from the area where it matters, they may sometimes remove all sensation from the waist downwards. That can make it less easy for a woman to know when to push, and so labour will be prolonged. They can also have some nasty side effects, like headaches, and it can take a while to recover from them properly.

Doctors can also use instruments called *forceps* in particularly difficult births, and these are exactly what they sound like – large, specially shaped tongs for grasping the baby's head and easing her out. Another instrument which is used for the same purpose is the *vacuum extractor*. In this device, a small cap is fitted to the baby's head and kept there by suction, again enabling the doctor to ease her out. And of course there's surgery, and we'll be looking at Caesareans – the surgical removal of a baby from the womb – a little further on as well.

In short, the critics say that birth in a modern hospital can seem more like the creation of Frankenstein's monster than the natural process by which a normal human baby is brought into the world. As one woman said to me, the contrast between the way a baby is begun and the way she's born could hardly be bigger! For with all these techniques and drugs there are machines, monitors to be strapped on to the labouring mother's stomach to see how she's getting on, winking lights and bleeping drip counters. There are the sometimes harsh lights and white walls of hospital architecture and people in gowns and masks and caps and rubber boots.

Is it any wonder that a lot of women find they don't enjoy it all very much?

Getting the birth you want

If that little gallery of horrors has completely put you off the whole idea of having a baby, I'm not surprised. "It's all so undignified," is what Sally had to say about it. The birth of our first child, Emma, was very much a hospital birth; poor Sally was 'semi-induced' (she was put on a drip to speed up her contractions, and at one time the drip was slowed down to put the brakes on as the staff weren't ready for the delivery). "I didn't feel that we had any control over what was happening, and that was a little frightening, to say the least," says Sally now. "But it was the indignity of it all that really got to me. Looking back it did make me feel very disappointed and depressed."

It's a proven fact that your experience of birth can be an important factor in determining whether or not you become seriously depressed afterwards. If you're very disappointed and upset by what happened to you during the birth, then that could be the start of a depression which might ruin the early part of parenthood – and those early days are tough enough as it is, anyway.

The good news is that there can be little doubt times *have* changed as far as birth is concerned, and things are still improving. In many countries the criticism levelled at the way birth has been handled has led to real improvements. Gradually, it seems, doctors and midwives are letting women have more say in how they give birth – and also letting nature take its course as far as possible.

More and more doctors are interested in the natural methods of childbirth, and are allowing women to get up and move around during their labours. This means for many women that birth is less technological and more relaxed than it was for their mothers – or even their older sisters.

But I don't want you to get the impression that all medical help in birth is interference and positively harmful. Many doctors say – quite rightly, too – that it's the medicalisation of childbirth which has helped to make it the safe experience it is today. Very few women suffer permanent damage or die in childbirth these days; in fact this sort of thing is so rare as to be considered extremely unusual. But it wasn't all that long ago that birth could be a very unsafe event for both mother and baby.

Many doctors would now agree with the critics of impersonal hospital methods that it's important for mothers to feel happy with what's going on. A relaxed, happy and confident mother is probably going to have an easier time – and that's going to make the midwife's and doctor's jobs that much easier as well. That means only using methods like induction and episiotomy when they're absolutely necessary, and sometimes they can be of great help – and also explaining to the mother (and her partner) *why* they're being used, so they can feel part of what's happening.

Here we come back to the importance of preparation. If you know what's likely to happen in birth, then you can talk to your doctor and midwife beforehand and tell them how you'd like to handle it. For example, you could tell them that you wanted to try and get through it without an episiotomy and ask them to ask *you* about it before it's done. You could ask them not to give you any painkillers until you ask for them, too. On the other hand, if you don't think you'll be able to cope with the pain just by having an active birth or doing breathing exercises, it's important to talk over what method of pain relief you'll want. It takes time to set up an epidural, for example – an anaesthetist has to be found, and it can't usually be done unless you book it beforehand.

The point is that if you feel you're in control and that the staff are *helping* you, rather than treating you as if you had no will or mind of your own, you're likely to get more out of the experience. In the end it's important to remember that it's *your* body and *your* child – and that you have a right to bring your baby into the world in the way which satisfies you, as far as that's possible. You have a choice, and it's one you should protect.

One result of the debate about birth today has been that many women would like to have their babies at home, rather than in hospital. There are many groups all over the world who believe that this should happen, and in some countries large numbers of women do have home births. Supporters of home birth say that birth in hospital can never be as relaxed and pleasant as birth at home; that hospitals are by their very nature impersonal.

But very few babies are born at home in Britain or America, and it's very rare for a first time mother to be allowed to give birth at home by her doctor. There are several reasons for this. First, now that most births happen in hospital, there aren't enough midwives to go out and help women give birth at home and in Britain, at least, it's a legal requirement to have a midwife at the birth. Second, most doctors are opposed to home birth because they say that the hospital is the only place where there are the right facilities to cope with emergencies.

The debate goes on, although it appears that the number of home births is growing. There's no doubt that most births are normal and straightforward, and could happen at home; but the doctors have a point too when they talk about potentially disastrous emergencies. One compromise has been to try and make hospitals more like homes, with comfortable furnishings in relaxed *birthing rooms* rather than stark, white surgical surroundings. The important thing to remember is that you even have a choice about where you give birth. It's not impossible for a first time mother to arrange for her baby to be born at home, although in many countries it can be difficult to persuade doctors and midwives to agree. Organisations exist to help women who want a home birth – and it may only need a certain amount of forcefulness. Any medical problem such as an illness, or any of the problems I have discussed which might make you a risk case, will certainly mean that the best place for you to have your baby is in hospital.

Your feelings

So how will you feel as all this is going on? In simple terms, you'll probably feel like you've never felt before, or will again. A first birth is an amazing, awe inspiring, terrifying and ecstatic experience. Everyone is unique, so your personal feelings during the birth of your child will be your own – but most people seem to go through the same gamut of feelings. It's like living an entire emotional life in a few hours. In short, it can be absolute magic.

You may feel nervous, worried or even panic stricken when labour starts. You may get annoyed or irritated at certain stages, and some women spend a lot of time cursing and swearing at their partners, the doctors and the midwives as a way of letting off steam. Some women say they'll never have sex again. Despair is another common feeling, especially if labour goes wrong or takes a long time. We've seen that women can feel disappointed at what happens to them, too.

A lot of women seem to feel taken over by a powerful force, something they can't do anything about; this is a feeling which comes particularly when they start to push in the second stage of labour, as the baby is about to be born. It's a primal, instinctive experience at that stage – something which has to happen, inevitably.

And then there's the huge relief which comes when the baby is finally born. That relief is mostly physical, of course; one woman said to me that at that last stage, giving birth felt like "sitting on the toilet and bringing the worst constipation of my life to an end. It was like passing a melon." I remember the look on Sally's face at that moment, each time; the relief was enormous once the baby was out. But there's an emotional relief in knowing that birth, this mighty, titanic experience, is almost over.

Both times Sally sat up immediately and had a look at the baby she had just delivered, who lay between her legs. I was there too, of course, watching in amazement, examining every inch, every tiny hair of this perfect little human being I'd just seen born, and who was still attached to her mother by the pulsing umbilical cord. For me – and all the men I've talked to about it have said virtually the same thing – that moment is almost indescribable. Each time I've experienced it I've burst into tears; and each time I've been reduced to almost complete speechlessness – something none of the people who know me can believe.

At any rate, the moment of birth is a vital one for the baby, too. Some babies actually cry as soon as they emerge into the world – which means they've taken their first independent breath. Many don't, and the first thing the medical staff are going to make sure of before the umbilical cord is cut is that the baby is breathing. Usually the baby's nasal passages and throat are blocked up with mucus, and perhaps some blood, and the midwife will probably clear her out to get her breathing. Babies are also covered in a cheesy substance called *vernix* and they can look very squashed up and ugly, and that can sometimes be a bit of a shock for the parents.

Once breathing is established, many hospitals these days operate a policy of laying the baby on the mother's stomach to allow both of them to come into skin contact as soon as possible. It's only fair, after all, that they should be allowed to meet at this moment – they've waited a long time for it. *Bonding* is very important, that process by which a relationship between mother and child begins to grow. The evidence shows that the sooner they can get into contact after birth, and the longer they can spend together, the better. Mothers who are separated from their babies after birth, for whatever reason, often find it harder to 'catch up' in bonding. It's important for fathers to have their chance to meet and get to know their babies, too, and I know that the moments when I held my newborn children in my arms for the first time were among the most memorable and important ones of my life.

Mothers are also encouraged these days to put their babies to the breast as soon as possible after birth. That's a pretty amazing sight – a newborn baby has an instinctive sucking reflex (remember all that thumb and finger sucking in the womb?), and it doesn't take much encouragement to get the baby sucking away strongly. Again, the evidence shows that the sooner the baby gets started on the breast, the easier it's going to be for both mother and child to keep breastfeeding going.

Anyway, there comes a time when the baby has to be taken away, however temporarily. The umbilical cord is clamped and cut (doctors believe this is painless for the baby), and the baby is then cleaned up to start with. She'll be weighed, and the circumference of her head and her length measured. These measurements are very important; they're the base line from which your baby's subsequent growth will be charted.

At some stage very soon after birth your baby will also be given a score out of ten, although she's not being marked in some sort of competition. It's a test called an *Apgar score*, and its purpose is to determine how healthy the baby is at birth – and whether she needs any special help. The baby is given marks for things like skin colour (which is a good indication of how well the blood is circulating), breathing, general appearance and so on. It's a handy way of assessing a baby quickly, and most children get a safe score of seven out of ten or more. Those with less than that may need help, and the lower the score, the more urgent the need for help.

Meanwhile, the mother is still busy – she'll probably be having the afterbirth delivered and, once this is over, the staff will begin to clean her up, too. Sometimes she'll get time to have a cup of tea or coffee and just relax in the knowledge that the worst part is over, and she's certain to have some more cuddles with her newborn baby, as will the new dad – if he hasn't dashed off to start telling the world he's got a son or daughter. It's these calm, quiet moments with the new baby that I always remember as the most joyful. You do things which seem silly at the time, but which – if you only knew it – are instinctive and universal. Things like counting the baby's fingers and toes to make sure they're all there, and doing a lot of talking to the baby, too; they're a very important part of that bonding process.

Some time after the birth a doctor will come and check the baby all over to make sure that she's healthy. This is a more in-depth check than the Apgar test, and will involve looking into the baby's mouth to check that there's no cleft palate, checking the head, the eyes, the ears, all the limbs and back and so on to make sure that there's no handicap, or defect of any kind. The mother will also be stitched if she's had an episiotomy or a tear, and then she'll be moved out of the delivery room and back to a ward where she can rest.

When things go wrong

Sadly, not all births go as well or end as joyfully as I've described. Various problems can happen to make things difficult, and these range from the relatively minor to the very serious. Every birth is unique, as your doctor will tell you, and you can never be sure that it's going to go as planned until it's all over.

First of all, labour can simply be very long or difficult. The position of the baby in the womb has a strong influence on this. That's why doctors or midwives check the baby's position throughout pregnancy. Babies do move about a lot in the womb, but your doctor will be hoping that your baby is in the right position in time for birth. The best position – that is, the one which will make birth easiest and safest – is for your baby to be head down in your pelvis (when she is said to have her head *engaged*), with the back of her head towards your front.

This is the commonest position for birth, and it means that the baby's head makes a sort of wedge shape, with her chin tucked down on to her chest. If a baby faces the other way, towards her mother's back – the head can't get into this shape, and this makes birth more difficult. The hardest births of all come when the baby is born brow first. In fact it's almost impossible for a baby to be born normally through the vagina in this way, and most of them have to be delivered by Caesarean.

Most people have heard of babies being born in the *breech* position, and this can make birth very difficult. All it means is that the baby hasn't turned to have her head facing downwards, and is born legs or buttocks first. Obviously this is more dangerous for mother and baby, and that's why many breech babies are born by Caesarean.

A Caesarean birth is the surgical removal of the baby from the womb. It is a technique which is used whenever a baby needs to be delivered quickly, or the mother has been labouring too long and is getting nowhere or can't deliver the baby normally for some reason. These days it is basically a very simple operation, although it is considered a major one. It does have its problems, though; for a start, a woman can feel very disappointed if she has to have an emergency Caesarean, and feel that she is missing out on giving birth. It also takes longer to recover from than from an ordinary birth, and if the mother has a general anaesthetic – that is, she is completely out for the operation – she may have problems with bonding or putting the baby to the breast in the early hours afterwards.

However, the problems aren't insuperable. Some women know they are going to have a Caesarean, and can prepare themselves for it. For example, it's sometimes found that a girl has a very small or narrow pelvis, and the doctors decide that the baby simply won't be able to come out. Obviously a Caesarean is then necessary – and that will probably mean she'll never be able to have a baby in the normal way, because once you've stopped growing, your pelvis isn't going to change shape any more. More and more women are having an epidural anaesthetic for their Caesareans, too; that means they're numb from the waist down and don't feel anything, but they're still awake and know what's going on. They're protected from the sight of anything unpleasant by a screen across their middles; and their partners can be with them too. It means they'll be able to see and hold their babies in those vital first few moments after birth.

Sometimes labour itself starts too early, and leads to the birth of a baby who is really too young and immature to survive. These babies – who may be very tiny indeed and who will probably need help with their breathing at the very least – are usually sent to special units where they can be looked after properly, *intensive* or *special care units for babies*. They may be placed in an *incubator*, a special sort of cot in which they can be monitored continuously and kept warm. These days doctors can even save some of the tiniest babies, and their skill in saving babies' lives is increasing day by day.

Unfortunately, some babies *are* born dead (this is called a *stillbirth*), and this is obviously very upsetting for parents. Parents can be very distressed after a miscarriage, and their depression can last for months; the same is true after a stillbirth. It's now known that parents grieve for their dead baby even if they've never known her alive, and need to be given time and help to cope with their grief. It's quite a rare occurrence these days, but it still does happen from time to time; and it's not something you can simply shrug off.

Something else which is going to have a major effect on a couple is the birth of a handicapped baby. Handicaps are many and varied. Some children are born with very minor handicaps, like a missing or extra finger, a slight deafness in an ear or a small birthmark. Others are terribly deformed or severely retarded. Many handicaps are the result of a fault in development during the baby's growth in the womb, while others are the result of external influences like German measles, a drug (Thalidomide was a case in point), or a difficult birth. Whatever the handicap, it comes as a terrible shock to find that the child you've been waiting for isn't as perfect as you'd hoped. For some parents this discovery comes immediately; for others it takes longer. Whenever it comes it turns the world upside down.

Thankfully, these days most parents of handicapped children are given more help than in the past. Much can also be done to minimise and even cure problems which would have caused a lifetime of misery in the old days. Hare lips and cleft palates can be surgically corrected, and club feet can be cured too. But for many children there is less hope; for those with spina bifida, for example, or cerebral palsy.

Again, it must be stressed that handicaps are uncommon these days, and *the vast majority of children are born normal*. Following the guidelines I laid down in Chapter 3 will also help to make sure that you avoid the tragedy of giving birth to a handicapped child. You should also remember that your antenatal check-ups are designed specifically to detect problems which can cause handicap as soon as possible so that they can be tackled effectively – so make sure you keep all your antenatal appointments.

Staying in hospital

In Britain – and the same is true of many other countries – most first time mothers spend a week or even ten days in hospital after the birth. One obvious reason for this is to make sure that both mother and baby are healthy and that everything is going well; if it isn't, then they're in the right place for something to be done about it.

In fact many women feel far better than they expected after birth. You'll feel quite sore, of course, and probably very tired as well. But you'll also feel suddenly slim now that your bump's gone, and for the first day or two you're more than likely to be riding high on the relief and joy you felt at the birth. You'll need to sleep, and being in hospital means that there will be expert help with the baby so that you can get your rest.

But mothers' feelings often take a sudden dip on the third or fourth day after the birth. In fact it's so common that it's considered positively normal. You might find yourself feeling very sensitive and irritable, as well as very depressed. Some women even spend the whole of the third or fourth day after the birth crying their eyes out.

There are various reasons for this. Firstly, most women have a sense of anticlimax. All the waiting of pregnancy is over, and the excitement and emotional release of the birth itself will have begun to wear off too. In short, you'll be coming down to earth; you'll be feeling the soreness more intensely as a result, and instead of being pleased simply to see that your bump has gone, you'll be depressed by the sight of the loose skin round your middle, and you'll be wondering if you'll ever make it back to your former shape. By now you may even be getting fed up with hospital food and routines – and simply want to go home.

Breastfeeding can play a part in 'the baby blues', too. If you've continued to put your baby to the breast since the birth, her sucking should have stimulated the milk glands to start working properly. I've already mentioned *colostrum*, the high protein milk a baby gets from the breast in the first few days of life. By day three or four this should have disappeared, the milk proper should be coming in, and breastfeeding should really be getting under way.

Breastfeeding is the natural way to feed your baby, as well as being the easiest and the best. But that doesn't mean it's always problem free. Many first time mothers need plenty of help and advice to get it going, and they can become very worried about whether they're getting it right. It's easy at this time to become very anxious and worked up about feeding; it is the baby's only way of getting any food, after all. If it's going badly — and anxiety won't help — it can lead to all sorts of problems, ranging from very sore nipples to very unhappy babies. Some women give up breastfeeding and start to bottle feed their babies, something which needn't be a disaster — but which can make you feel very guilty. There's also the problem of suppressing your milk supply if you don't breastfeed, and that can mean several days of sore and swollen breasts.

It's also important to remember that a woman's body goes through some dramatic changes after birth, too. For a start, the womb begins to shrink back to its pre-pregnant size. Breastfeeding helps this process along; the baby's sucking stimulates the production of a hormone which makes the womb contract. In fact this can be quite painful. Sally said that it was one of the biggest surprises of this time for her. "As I breastfed Emma in the early days in hospital, I could feel my womb contracting. Nobody told me it would be so painful, though. It was almost like going through labour again."

The hormone levels in a woman's body also change dramatically in the early days after the birth, as the body begins to get back to normal. The levels of some hormones in the system drop to one hundredth or even one thousandth of their level during pregnancy, and this obviously has something to do with the fluctuations in mood a woman might experience. Some women find their swings of mood to be more of a problem than just being fed up — one moment they can be ecstatic, and the next, terribly depressed. For many mothers there's an element of disappointment at this time. Babies can look very ugly; they can be red and wrinkled and have odd lumps and bumps, and even have misshapen heads, all the result of the pressures of birth – and all quite normal. Some babies look a little yellowish, a sign of *jaundice*, which is quite common and generally nothing to worry about. Some have big ears or sticky eyes. All babies have a stump where their umbilical cords were cut, and this can look quite unpleasant, with a lot of dried blood and a clamp still in position. In these early days, what a newborn baby fills her nappy with also has to be seen to be believed – it's a black-green substance called *meconium* which has been in the intestines throughout pregnancy. Some baby girls frighten the lives out of their mothers by bleeding into their nappies. Sometimes hormones from the mother get across the placenta into the baby's system just before birth, and stimulate the baby's tiny womb to have a period. The same hormones can even make a little baby's nipples start to produce milk.

In short, a new mother is presented with a baby who might look very unlike the babies in the commercials on television; a real, crying, excreting, urinating, ugly little living doll with a will of her own. It's no wonder that you might have a few negative feelings towards this little creature, right from the very beginning. The problem is that most of us feel we should love our babies without question, and that negative feelings are somehow abnormal. The pressure to feel this way is particularly intense for young mothers.

In a survey quoted by *Parents* magazine in Britain, a large number of young, first time mothers were asked during their pregnancies what they expected to feel towards their babies when they were born. A staggering 81 per cent of them said they thought they would feel an immediate sense of love. The same women were asked whether they had actually felt that way after the birth – and only 37 per cent said they did. The result for many of these mothers was simple – they felt guilty, and few of them felt that they could talk about it to anybody; which meant that they just had to suppress the feelings, instead of getting them out in the open. Suppressed feelings have a tendency to fester and come out later in one way or another.

The important word in this context is *time*. Remember that you need time to meet and get to know your new child, and that if you let it happen, you will develop feelings of love. For some parents they come quite soon, even immediately – and they continue to grow throughout their children's lives. There's no need to expect too much from yourself at the beginning – and there's certainly no need to feel guilty. These early days in hospital can be very confusing, very emotional and very strange. At the bottom of all these feelings is the knowledge that the biggest job of your life has begun – and you're bound to wonder whether you'll be able to cope or not. You will – but you've yet to prove it to yourself. Then again, you might be one of the parents who falls in love with their baby immediately, and thinks she's the most perfect, most beautiful baby in the world. If you do, then that's all to the good.

The advantage of being in hospital at this time is that at least there are people around to help you. There are the doctors and midwives, for example, and it's important not to be afraid to ask about anything which might be worrying you. There are also the other mothers, some of whom will have delivered second or subsequent babies – and they're marvellous sources of advice. You may even know some of them from the antenatal clinic or your classes. It's worth building on any friendships you make in hospital, too – people who are going through the same sort of experiences can often help each other with advice and support.

Time to go home

Hospitals aren't perfect, though, and you may feel yourself becoming increasingly impatient to get home. This time is often particularly difficult for fathers, too. After the involvement in the pregnancy and the thrill of being at the birth, they may suddenly find themselves reduced to the status of visitors. Even though many hospitals have now extended their visiting hours so that fathers can spend a lot more time with their new families, it can still be a period when you feel isolated and left out. I know I did; it was very frustrating to come home to an empty house after visiting my wife and new baby daughter. I felt as if I hadn't really started being a father yet.

But the big day comes eventually. The doctor usually comes round to check that both mother and baby are fit enough to go home. Then the doors of the hospital are open, and it's time to take the biggest step in your life – the one that leads into the total responsibility of parenthood. From now on you're on your own.

Part 3. **Beginning to be a parent**

7. Home with your baby

SOMEONE once described the early days of parenthood to me as an earthquake. I couldn't see what she meant at first, but then the more I thought about it, the clearer it became – and I began to see that it was a very appropriate description. When that tiny baby makes her entrance into your life, however well prepared you are, everything about your existence is shaken, rattled, disturbed and generally tossed into the air. It all settles down – eventually – but nothing is in exactly the same place as it used to be, or will ever be quite the same again. From that moment on, life is definitely going to be different.

The actual experience of looking after your own baby *will* come as a shock. If you have any rosy illusions about it, now's the time when they will be shattered. Look at it this way. Imagine that you have been learning to drive a car. You've read all about cars and how they work. You've read about changing gear and signalling, overtaking and road courtesy, engines and accelerators, clutches and steering wheels. You've looked at pictures of cars and pored over diagrams and charts. You've talked to other people about their cars, and you've even been for a ride in one – once. You've seen lots of cars in the streets and you've even played with a toy car once or twice.

But there's one thing you've never done – you've never actually put the theory into practice and driven a real car.

Then you go for your driving test, and to your horror, you discover that you're expected to get into a car and drive it round the traffic filled streets. And what's worse, you're not supposed to make any mistakes at all!

If you can imagine all that, then you might get some idea of how it feels in the early days of parenthood. It's a time of chaos and seemingly total panic; a time of sudden responsibility, self doubt, fear, worry and stress. It can also be a time of great joy as well as very rapid learning and personal growth. The important point to keep in mind, as with almost every aspect of becoming a parent, is that you have to understand the problems if you want to enjoy the good things of this time as well. For now is the time when theory really does have to be translated into practice – and a baby is a lot more difficult to manage than a car!

A 24-hour-a-day job

Newborn babies are very, very demanding creatures. "I never realised just how demanding a newborn baby could be," one mother told me, "until I had to start coping with my own. It really is a 24-hour-a-day job. It seems at first as if there's never any relief at all."

Their needs are simple. A baby wants milk and sleep; the first she gets from you, and the second she takes whenever she needs it. If she's hungry she'll wake up and cry – and she'll keep crying until her hunger is satisfied, when she'll probably drift off to a contented sleep. At this stage she also has absolutely no conception of day or night. That means she's just as likely to want feeding in the middle of the night as she does in the middle of the day. She won't care if you've only just gone to sleep; if she's hungry, she'll cry to be fed.

"Before you have your baby people talk about broken nights and loss of sleep," one woman said. "If you're like me, you'll think that it can't possibly be as bad as they say it is. But when you're actually going through it yourself, you begin to wonder if you'll ever live to see your child's first birthday."

Newborn babies are also extremely messy. They have no manners, and are often sick, usually over the person who's holding them – and that's you. They also have no control over their bladders or bowels, which means they empty their contents whenever they're full, and wherever they happen to be at the time. That's why they have to wear nappies – and nappies have to be changed. I've already described the sight of the meconium in a baby's nappy during the first couple of days. By the baby's second week, she should be passing motions which look a slightly more normal colour – light brown or yellowish brown. They're likely to be very liquid, and that's because babies' diets at this stage are all liquid. That doesn't stop the nappies looking extremely unpleasant and smelling.

Our daughter Helen developed a habit when she was very young which shows just how messy a baby can be. We used to dress her in tiny all-in-one suits which had poppers all up the front. Anyway, no matter how well we put her nappy on, or how carefully we checked to see that her plastic pants covered it, Helen always seemed to manage to overflow. We lost count of the number of times we picked her up out of her cot to find one leg – sometimes both – of her all-in-one suit filled to the brim. And there is nothing worse to have to face in the middle of the night than *that*.

Tiny babies can be very worrying, too. It takes a while for the umbilical cord stump to wither up and fall off. It will bleed sometimes, and you'll find yourself dabbing at it very gently, terrified that you're causing your baby a lot of pain. It also takes time simply to get used to handling a baby. They're very light, but their heads are much the heaviest and floppiest part of them, so they need to be supported in this area when you pick them up. But there isn't a parent alive who hasn't picked up her baby in the wrong way in the early days and seen the head flop back. It can make your stomach churn with panic as you think you've broken your baby's neck. She'll probably fling all her limbs out in the *startle reflex*. That will frighten the life out of you – and make you feel very guilty. But babies are, a lot tougher than they look.

Bath time seems to be a particularly worrying event for many first time parents. Babies are very messy little creatures, and they need to be kept clean for various reasons. The main one is, of course, that life is more pleasant for you if your baby is clean most of the time. Babies left in dirty nappies for too long may also develop nappy rash, and that can make their bottoms very sore. With this in mind, most parents are advised to give their babies a daily bath.

These days you can buy specially designed baby baths which help to make life easier. There's also a definite technique for bathing a tiny baby, which involves making sure you've got all you need close to hand – and that means talc, powders, creams, nappies, towels, clothes and so on – and making sure you take your time. The water has to be the right temperature, too – not too hot or cold. As you bath the baby, you have to support her head with one hand and wash her with the other. Some babies love it, others loathe it and scream continually throughout, something which can send your blood pressure through the roof. Bath time is also fraught with all sorts of tiny things which can worry the life out of you until you get used to doing them – things like cutting your baby's fingernails to make sure she doesn't scratch herself, and cleaning the corners of her eyes.

Continual panic

So there you are, the proud parents of a brand new baby, at home together for the first time. I've never forgotten my personal experience of those days, and I don't think anybody ever does. In fact, just to make sure that we didn't forget, we made some notes as it was happening. I've sifted through them to produce what you'll read in this section; the average day of a couple with a two-week-old baby, which was filled with almost continual activity – and panic.

5 am Emma woke up for her first feed of the day. It only seemed like five minutes ago that she was having her last feed of yesterday, but then babies don't know the meaning of the word mercy. Sally got up to her, and I went to the kitchen to make us both a cup of tea. Emma wouldn't settle for a while after the feed, but did eventually. We slept fitfully until 6.30 when she woke up again, had a nappy change and another feed. Decided to get up.

7 am Hurried breakfast. Emma asleep.

8.15 am Bath time. It seemed to take ages to get everything together, but it was worth it. Emma really enjoyed her bath, so we took a long time over it. But then we panicked because we thought she was getting too cold. Another feed. She filled her nappy for the first time that day just after a clean one was put on, so she had to be changed again. After all her exertions, she slept quite soundly.

10.45 am Emma woke crying for another feed and nappy change. She was sick on the carpet over my shoulder this time, but went to sleep quite quickly.

12.30 pm Emma slept on, so it was time to try and grab a quick lunch before she woke up – which she did, just as our sandwiches and coffee were ready. More feeding and nappy changing. It was almost as if she could tell we wanted her to go back to sleep – she didn't, and cried for a while. The crying ended when she filled her nappy again.

2.00 pm The midwife called to see if everything was OK, and stayed for a cup of tea. Emma stayed asleep.

3.00 pm Emma woke for another quick feed and nappy change.

3.30 pm First visitor of the day – my sister called with her children after picking them up from school. They wanted to see the new baby, who was still awake. All the noise and attention kept her crying for a while, but a feed soon put her back to sleep.

4.30 pm Sister and her children went – neighbours dropped in. Emma stayed resolutely asleep, refusing to wake up for even the loudest 'coochie-coo'.

5.15 pm Another brief feed and nappy change.

7.00 pm Time for some dinner – but I still hadn't washed up the breakfast or lunch things because I'd been talking to all our visitors. Emma woke up for a very brief feed.

10.00 pm We got our dinner without being disturbed, and managed to sit comatose in front of the television while Emma slept soundly in her carrycot. Then she woke up for a feed. It was a long one, and we took great care to make sure she was clean and comfortable for bed in the hope that she would sleep longer. But we knew she would be awake in a few hours.

10.30 pm Emma fast asleep. Sally went to bed, exhausted, and I followed soon after, once I'd tidied up and done a whole day's washing up at once. Tomorrow I'll have to do some washing – we're running out of clothes.

2.00 am Emma wakes for her night feed, and we both feel really dreadful. Sally changes the nappy and feeds her, while I watch. I couldn't get back to sleep even when Sally and Emma were snoring, though – I knew I was going to be woken up again in a few hours!

Looking through these notes brings back all sorts of memories. I can remember the tiredness, and the feeling that

I'd never been so tired in all my life. I can remember working out that one little baby was going through almost a dozen nappies in 24 hours, 84 a week, and we'd only bought two dozen – so you can imagine how much washing we were having to do. I can remember cleaning out the nappies before they were put into the wash, and rinsing them through. I remember thinking that I couldn't believe a lot of the things I was doing. And I remember being convinced through it all that I was a *terrible* parent, a real disaster in the fatherhood stakes.

A skill to be learned

For some reason, many of us think that we should be good parents right from the word go, that we should instinctively know how to handle our own babies and look after them without any help or advice. It's simply not that way, though. That's what I wanted to emphasise at the beginning of this chapter by talking about learning to drive a car.

There *are* some instinctive things about being a parent, but it's vital to remember that in those early weeks, you and your baby are total strangers to each other. She doesn't know you and you don't know her. Coming home from hospital with you is as much of a shock for her as it is for you. You don't, and couldn't possibly know what she wants all the time, and what will satisfy her every need. You've got a pretty good idea that she needs milk, sleep and some cuddles, but you have to *learn* from her when is the right time to give her which – and how much she needs. All that takes time.

We tend to think of learning as something that children do, but when it comes to the early days of parenthood, the *baby* is the teacher. You're struggling to learn about her, and also about yourself; and together you have to work out a way of living together. In the end, that's what it's all about; these early days of parenthood represent a real transition in life, one in which you have to make major adjustments. Getting things right at this time will make dealing with what follows a lot easier.

Learning plays a part in virtually every area of parenthood, and one of the delights of being a parent for me is that I learn something new every day. Sometimes it's about myself, sometimes about my children; but whichever it is, I'm learning all the time. What I'm saying is that you don't leap into action as a fully fledged parent from day one – you have to learn how to do it. You have to learn how to fold a nappy, for example, and your first efforts will probably be a disaster. You'll have to learn all sorts of things as they grow up, and the process never really ends.

Unfortunately you don't get much time at the beginning, and you certainly won't have much energy. The early days often seem to be a blur, when everything happens at once. As you can see from the average day I've outlined above, you're busy all the time. In between nappy changes and feeds you're probably trying to tidy up, deal with the endless stream of visitors a newborn baby seems to attract, or simply catch up on your rest. Mothers will still feel sore up to three or four weeks after the birth, too, and both parents will be struggling with a complete set of new emotions and thoughts about their lives. On top of that you'll probably feel very keen to do the right thing all the time – and you're bound to feel that it's a serious business.

I remember waking up in the middle of the night when Emma was only a couple of weeks old. As you've seen, that wasn't unusual. But on this particular night, I couldn't hear any of the usual snuffling, breathing noises coming from the cot at the end of our bed – and I panicked. I shot out of bed in the dark and crashed into Sally, who was already bending over the cot, desperately listening to make sure Emma was still breathing, and terrified at the same time in case she woke her up. We both had to laugh; and of course Emma did wake up; and stayed awake for the next couple of hours. Most of the other parents I know would admit that they too have got up in the middle of the night just to check on their newborn babies, even if they've already been up half a dozen times. You do it because your baby's important to you and you feel totally responsible – in other words, you *worry*.

In the end, it's those feelings which make the early days of parenthood so difficult. You realise that your baby's completely dependent on you; and you worry that you're not doing the right thing. You worry about whether she's taking enough milk, whether she's warm enough, whether you're normal in the way you feel – in fact, you worry about everything. "I didn't know there was so much to worry about," one father said to me. "I got to the stage where I was worried if I wasn't worrying about something."

Feeding your baby

Most first time parents spend a lot of time worrying about one thing above all – and that's feeding. Whether you breastfeed or bottle feed, you'll find that you're very concerned about it sometimes, and it's easy to see why, as it's your baby's sole means of gaining the nourishment she needs.

Small babies can only take food in the form of milk, and there are two ways of providing it. There's the old fashioned way, the way which is as old as the human race – breastfeeding. And there's also the newer method, one which has only really taken off during this century – and that's bottle feeding. In the latter, the milk which is used isn't human breast milk, it's cows' milk which has been modified to make it more like breast milk. It's also sold in powdered form, and has to be made up with water before it can be given to a baby in a specially made bottle with a rubber teat.

Bottle feeding has become so common in this century that people don't think of it as being odd any more. But it's a very odd phenomenon indeed, if you think about it. Human women have breasts, and almost all women are physically capable of producing milk for their babies. So why should they give them artificial milk in a bottle? There are no other animals who do the same, after all.

It's hard to say why bottle feeding became so popular. Some people think it was part of the general move away from natural things that we've seen in this century. Most of the food we eat is processed, refined or changed in some way; few of us eat really natural foods. Few of us live in the country or are close to nature in any way. Perhaps it seemed right that babies in cities should be given artificial milk. It also has something to do with being more scientific about bringing up our children.

Supporters of bottle feeding in the past claimed that it was better because you could see – and control – the quantity and the 'quality' of the food the baby was getting.

But there's one theory about the rise of bottle feeding which I think says it all. I talked earlier on about society's attitude to women. Women are supposed to want to have children, and are encouraged to think of themselves as mothers. But male-dominated society also encourages women to look after their figures, to stay attractive, to be seductive and so on. That's why I talked about the problems some women experience during pregnancy. You spend most of your life buying clothes and cosmetics to make you look attractive and going on diets to stay slim, but then to have a baby you have to become 'fat and ugly'.

At the same time, you can see a lot of breasts in modern society. In 'girlie' magazines, national newspapers, books, on television and in films, on posters and hoardings and even on packets and wrappers, breasts are everywhere. And more often than not they're young, firm and not spurting breast milk. The theory says that girls are brought up to see their breasts as ways of attracting men, as part of their sexual attraction, and not as a means of feeding their babies. Breastfeeding, to many women, seems almost disgusting – "Like being a cow," as one woman put it to me. Many girls are also worried that breastfeeding will ruin the look and shape of their breasts permanently. With all this in mind, some women simply don't like the idea of breastfeeding and its close, physical intimacy – and so they bottle feed.

But this is another area where times are changing. There's evidence that more and more women are turning away from bottle feeding and back to the more natural way. That can only be a good thing – for a number of reasons. The first of these is, quite simply, that breast milk is the best food for a human baby, because it's specifically designed for *her*.

First of all, breast milk has all the right nutrients in the right proportions. It also passes on immunities to common infections from mother to child, which helps to keep a baby healthy in the early months. Breastfed babies also tend to be free of *allergies*. An allergy is an inappropriate reaction by the body to a substance which is harmless; hay fever sufferers are allergic to pollen, for example, and coming into contact with too much of it produces the symptoms of a cold – runny nose, sneezes and so on. In recent years there has been much research into allergies, and it's been discovered that cows' milk products are a very common cause of them – especially in babies.

An allergy to cows' milk or any other dairy product can cause a number of symptoms in a baby. It can cause *eczema*, a distressing, itchy skin condition. It's also been linked to a condition called *hyperactivity*. Hyperactive children don't sleep very much, behave badly, have terrible tantrums and swings of mood, and generally drive their parents to the end of their tether. It's been found that sometimes simply removing milk products or other substances to which they might be allergic from their diets changes them into much calmer, more pleasant – and happier – children.

Breastfeeding is also by far the easiest way of feeding a baby. Bottles of milk have to be prepared. The bottles and teats have to be kept scrupulously sterile, the milk has to be mixed and heated (although most babies won't mind taking it cold) – all of which takes time. Fiddling around with teats and bottles at two in the morning while your baby is screaming for her feed can make life very difficult. Breastfeeding can be so simple, in contrast – it's simply a matter of bringing baby and breast into contact.

But it isn't always that simple. As with every part of becoming a parent, it will be easier if you decide positively to feed your baby in this way, and then take steps to make it as easy for you as possible. That means looking after your breasts in the way I recommended in Chapter 5. It means finding out about breastfeeding from people and organisations who can help you, like your doctor, midwife and health visitor. There are also several good books on the subject, details of which you'll find in the list at the end of this book. The more you know about the theory, the less surprised you'll be about the reality.

At any rate, two things will help to make breastfeeding easier once you get started, and that's making sure you stay relaxed, and asking the advice of someone who knows about it as soon as you hit a problem. It's easy to say that you should stay relaxed; mothers often become very worried about the baby not getting enough milk. It's been found that anxiety hinders the milk supply and upsets the baby, who senses that her mother is worried and unhappy. This in turn makes the mother more worried, and pretty soon she's in a vicious circle of more worry and less milk, until finally she gives up and puts the baby on the bottle.

Breastfeeding is, however, the classic example of the supply and demand system. The more the breasts are stimulated by the baby's sucking, the more milk they'll produce. That's why doctors now recommend that you should feed a baby *on demand*, that is, whenever she's hungry. In that way, she'll stimulate the breasts to provide as much as she needs, and she'll feed until she's satisfied. There's no point in making a very young baby wait to be fed as mothers used to be advised; she'll only cry until she gets what she wants. Very small babies might want to feed every hour or two in the first few weeks of life. After a longer gap they'll take more, after a shorter gap they'll take less; but if you relax and let the baby lead the way, she'll get exactly what she needs.

There's also a definite technique to breastfeeding, and this is where you might need some advice to begin with. The baby should get the whole of the nipple in her mouth, including the darker area – called the areola – around it. The nipple should go a long way back in her mouth. If she isn't *latched on* properly in this way, her sucking can make your nipples very sore. You also need to hold your baby comfortably, and this might mean sitting in a comfortable chair with cushions under your arm. Most mothers find their own most comfortable position. Young babies tend to fall asleep during their feeds, although some may keep sucking while they doze. You should never pull your baby off the nipple, either; it's best to insert a finger between her mouth and the nipple and ease her off gently – pulling her off will just hurt and lead to soreness.

It's important to seek advice if any problems should crop up, though. Some women do get sore breasts, and even *cracked nipples* – which can be very painful indeed. You can get an infection in the breast, which might lead to a *breast abscess*, otherwise known as *mastitis*. These problems can be dealt with, and women can even manage to keep breastfeeding through them. It's possible to express breast milk by hand and give it to a baby in a bottle; there are special breast pumps and bottles for this purpose. This not only helps when there's a problem, it can also allow fathers or babysitters to feed the baby while Mum gets a break or catches up on her sleep.

It is worth breastfeeding your baby for however long you can manage it. When it's going well, most women would say there's nothing like it. There's a warmth and intimacy about this natural way of feeding which helps in the development of a relationship between mother and child; all that close skin contact helps in this context. The milk for a feed comes into a breast through what's known as the *let-down reflex*. Some women feel this when they pick their babies up, while others feel it as soon as they hear their babies start to cry.

There are a couple of other advantages in breastfeeding which few people know about until it happens to them. The first is that the hormones you need in your system to keep your breasts producing milk stop you ovulating as a side effect – and that means you won't have any periods. This only lasts so long as you're fully breastfeeding on demand, and as soon as your baby starts missing out on feeds as she gets older, your periods are likely to return. Not every woman looks on this as an advantage, although many I've spoken to do.

Of course, not ovulating means you can't become pregnant, and that means breastfeeding fully on demand does constitute a natural form of contraception. However, it's not a reliable one, because you have no way of telling when your ovulation starts again. That's why many doctors recommend that you use some form of contraception when you resume your sex life after the birth, even though breastfeeding may protect you to a large extent. Still, the advantage is that if you do use some form of contraception, you can be pretty sure that you won't become pregnant while you're breastfeeding – and it's a good back up in case of mistakes!

There's been a lot of talk about the other benefits of breastfeeding in recent years, with the result that very many

7. Home with your baby

women – probably the majority – start off intending to feed their babies in this way. Many give up after a few weeks or a month, but many also manage to keep going. There's no need to set a time limit to how long you feed your baby. Even when your child starts to take solid food – which usually happens at around four months – she'll still enjoy sucking, as much for the comfort and warmth it brings as for the milk. Some women feed their babies for a year or even longer.

A new problem has arisen, though, because so much emphasis is placed on how good breastfeeding is for babies. Some women simply find the idea repugnant and don't want to breastfeed. Others try and don't like it or find that they can't keep it going, maybe because they have a problem like a cracked nipple. But whatever their reason for not breastfeeding, women like these can feel guilty or feel that they've failed their babies in some way because 'breast is always best'.

That's the message from doctors and baby care experts these days, and I must say that I do feel 'breast is best'. There are very, very few women who are truly, *physically* unable to breastfeed in the sense that their breasts don't work properly as other women's do. Many women find that they *can't* breastfeed because they don't like the idea; they find it difficult, or they have one of the problems I've mentioned; all of which are perfectly understandable reasons for not breastfeeding. But it's important to remember that many, many women who don't breastfeed are capable of it given the right help and advice. I believe that we should encourage as many women as possible to breastfeed, for their own sake as well as for their babies.

Nevertheless, I heartily disapprove of the idea that women who bottle feed should feel guilty about it. There are women who don't want to or can't breastfeed, and for many years by far the majority of babies got their milk from bottles and not from breasts. Sally gave up breastfeeding Emma at four months and switched to bottles, mostly out of anxiety that she didn't have enough milk. With Helen and Thomas she's been much more relaxed and has had more than enough milk. But I know just how anxious parents can get about feeding, and it's that anxiety which can often cause problems. One good thing about bottle feeding for us was that it meant I could help out more at feeding times – which was a real bonus for both of us, even though it meant a few late nights for me!

If you do bottle feed, it's important to make sure you follow the rules. The rules for bottle feeding are simple. Keep the bottles and teats clean and sterile; you can buy special kits which come complete with a set of feeding bottles for this purpose. Always obey the instructions on the packet of milk powder – never add more powder than it says. Doing this might just make your baby fat, and fat babies turn into fat adults. Feed your baby on demand, just as if she was breastfed, and don't try to force her to take more than she wants at any one time. And make feeds a time for cuddles and 'conversations' with your baby. It's at feeds that you really build your relationship with a young baby.

Getting your figure back

One thing you're bound to be thinking about in these early days is getting your figure back. It's perfectly possible to restore your figure to almost exactly the same proportions as it was before you became pregnant. Again, breastfeeding helps – it uses up some of the extra fat you put on during pregnancy, and therefore gets rid of it more quickly. But you'll still have loose skin round your middle, and perhaps some extra weight in other areas, and the only way to get rid of all this is through exercise and sensible eating.

It's worth stressing that you shouldn't go on a crash or starvation diet at this time simply to get rid of some extra weight. If you've eaten sensibly through your pregnancy you shouldn't need to, and one thing you do need is plenty of energy to cope with the extra demands of these early days of parenthood. If you're breastfeeding it's especially important to make sure you eat a good balanced diet. Your baby's milk and the nutrients it contains is made of what you eat – so she's dependent on your diet as much as you are.

Many mothers – especially those who don't put on too much weight during pregnancy – find that the extra weight disappears fairly quickly anyway. All the hard work which goes with having a baby soon burns off those calories! Exercises help to tone up and tighten loose skin and muscles, and your doctor or midwife will probably give you some directions for these. Details of such exercises can also be found in some of the books I've recommended at the end of this book. But again, it's important not to overdo it. Doing frantic aerobics two or three weeks after the birth is only going to exhaust you – and may even make you ill. Your doctor will advise you to take your time, and you should certainly never do any exercises which hurt at this stage. Why not give yourself a target? Sally gave herself six months to get back into her jeans, and made it before the deadline each time! If you look after your breasts by wearing a good support bra during the time you're breastfeeding, they should stay in good shape. Something else many women worry about is their vagina. "I was convinced that having a baby would mean my vagina would become loose and floppy," one woman said. "I just couldn't see how things could turn out otherwise. After all, a big thing like a baby coming through such a small passage much stretch it completely out of shape, I thought."

She was pleased to discover that she was wrong. The vagina is a very elastic organ, and most women find that it's back to normal within a couple of weeks after birth. Most women have a heavy period after birth in the early weeks anyway – it's the womb clearing out all the debris and thick lining which has supported the placenta and the baby throughout the pregnancy, and it's called the *lochia*.

How soon your vagina recovers depends, of course, on what sort of battering it took during the birth. Tears and cuts take a while to heal, and you could find that you're sore for several weeks. It has been known, as well, for an episiotomy to be stitched up wrongly; in this case you might be in a lot of pain. If you are still in pain after a few weeks, it's worth asking your doctor to check that everything is all right. Most women are given a thorough check at six weeks after the birth when problems like this sometimes come to light.

It's worth taking some steps to tone up the muscles in that area, which doctors call the *pelvic floor*. The muscles in question are called the *pubococcygeus muscles*. You can feel these muscles in operation (I'm only talking to female readers here!) if you try to stop the flow while you're urinating. Tightening and relaxing them is the way to tone them up – and doing this constitutes a set of pelvic manoeuvres known to doctors as *Kegal exercises*. You can do them at any time of day, anywhere – and they really do tighten up the vagina.

Of course, once your vagina has recovered fully, you'll be able to resume your sex life. It's wise to take this very easily at first, and many women wait until they get the final go-ahead from the doctor at the six weeks check-up. It can be a little uncomfortable at first, but everything should be back to normal by six weeks after the birth at the latest. If it isn't, ask your doctor for his advice.

Your relationship

That doesn't mean to say that things are going to be exactly the same as they used to be; they're not. Many young couples with small babies find that they simply don't have the time or energy to make love as often as they used to, and also find that they don't enjoy it as much as before.

It's not very surprising. It's hard to be romantic when you're completely exhausted and when you're waiting for the baby to cry for her next feed all the time. Breastfeeding mums are likely to go to bed with their support bras on, especially when they're producing a lot of milk. You soon find out that any pressure on the breasts when they're full can produce spurts of milk – and that can dampen even the most ardent couple's passion!

In fact it can take many months for a couple's sex life to recover anywhere near fully. It just seems very often that it's the last thing on a list of priorities, and therefore doesn't get much attention. It also suffers because of the sort of attitudes society drums into us from a very young age. It's a fact that we tend to see parenthood and sex as two things which don't go together. All the images in commercials, magazines, films and television of sex feature young people, people without children; society tends to assume that mums and dads *aren't* sexy, and probably shouldn't be.

A lot of women therefore find that they don't feel very keen on the idea of sex any more now that they've got a baby. Some men also find it hard to think of their wives as people with sexual needs and desires any more. There's also the problem of the jealousy which can sometimes creep into a relationship in these early days. I've said that men can feel jealous of their babies before they're even born, and that feeling can grow after the birth. Some women don't have much time or energy to spare for their partners, and devote all their attention to their babies, leaving Dad to feel alienated and left out. Some women feel the same if their partners take too much notice of the baby.

All of these feelings can sour a relationship at a time when both partners need each other's strength and support to cope with all the stresses and strains. Many couples say that their level of satisfaction with their marriages drops after the birth of a first baby. Those stresses put both parents under pressure; and any pressure is bound to widen any cracks which there might be in the relationship, and we all know that every relationship has its weak points.

The problem is that very often both partners feel they shouldn't mention any negative feelings they have towards each other or the baby. It's best to get anything like that out into the open and talk it over; silence means brooding and resentment, and that's bad in any relationship at any stage.

Hard as it may be, it's vital for you to think of your relationship at this time. I've talked in this chapter about learning to be a parent. You also have to learn to live with each other as parents, and you're going to discover many things about your partner as you both cope with what's happening to you. What you need to remember is that your relationship is going to need some adjusting too.

Many men these days take time off work to be with their partners in the early weeks of parenthood. In some countries they're actually given *paternity leave* which is paid time off to spend with their families at such a crucial period.

But these countries are in the minority, and for most men it's a question of paid holiday or unpaid sick leave. But however difficult it is to arrange, it's very important for a father simply to *be there* if he can, in those first few weeks.

It's at this time that most young fathers begin the process of learning to be a parent. Most first time mothers will have spent a week or ten days in hospital while their partners languish at home. Fathers therefore have to do some catching up. Remember too that most boys and men aren't brought up to think of themselves as parents, or to see themselves changing nappies and getting up in the middle of the night to see to a crying baby. The shock of having a real live baby about the house is probably even worse for some men, and if they're going to take a share in bringing up their children, they have to make a special effort in those early days. The evidence shows that men who are interested and involved in their partners' pregnancies and who are at the birth get off to a flying start. But even they need some help.

The problem is simple. Their partners will have had time to develop some confidence at least in handling and looking after their babies. It's very easy – especially at times of pressure, such as in the middle of the night – for the more confident and experienced partner to do everything for the sake of speed. Mothers sometimes lose patience with their partners' clumsy efforts to change a nappy, and muscle in; their partners lose any confidence they might have had, don't gain any experience, and so leave basic child care increasingly to 'mother'.

It has to be said that though more men try these days, it's still a proven fact that babies are looked after most of the time by their mothers. Even where both partners work and the baby is looked after by a childminder or is in a nursery, it's been found that in the evenings and at weekends, mothers do more nappy changing and feeding, and so on. This needn't be so. Apart from the fact that men can't breastfeed, there's no instinctive difference between men and women when it comes to looking after children. Men can learn to change nappies just as well as women; men can be just as good at being a parent, sometimes better. All you need is the right attitude – and some time to learn.

Making a particular effort in the early days will also help to strengthen the relationship between partners. The more a man and woman share every part of looking after their new baby, the closer they're likely to be. It can be a difficult time for fathers; some men feel as if they can never do anything right. Their partners' moods swing from high to low, they're always tired or seeing to the baby, and sex is the last item on the list. It may mean being extra sensitive to your partner's needs until she is feeling more in control of what's happening to her. It's definitely important not to 'opt out' of looking after the baby, though, and to try and get as involved as you can.

Making time

Whatever your situation, the most important thing to remember about these early days and weeks of parenthood is that you need *time*. You need time to learn, you need time to make adjustments, you need time to cope with the massive shock that having a baby really is.

Nobody ever seems to get enough time, but you can make it easier for yourself simply by not expecting too much. If you expect too much of your baby, if you expect too much of yourself, there will be only one result; disappointment. It's far better to be realistic – and even a little pessimistic. For example, as I said, give yourself six months – or even a year – to get your figure back to its pre-pregnancy condition. If you don't bother to try you won't be very happy. If you try too hard and give yourself three months, you'll probably make yourself unhappy (and maybe ill), and if you do as I suggest you'll probably make it within the deadline and feel very pleased with yourself indeed. The same method can be used with any part of the experience of becoming a parent.

It's also important to take any short cuts, cut any corners and do anything easy at such a time of intense pressure, especially in those early weeks. Don't worry about housework or doing the washing; don't try to cook cordon bleu meals. It's important to eat good, wholesome food, as it is at any time of life; but it doesn't matter if the food's very simple for a while and easy to prepare. The most vital task of this period is for all of you to get to know each other and get used to living together – and that means mother, father and baby. Nothing should be allowed to get in the way of that process. It isn't just a baby who is born at this time; a whole new family is born as well.

Don't be afraid to ask for any help or advice either. In fact it's highly likely that your doctor or midwife or some other professional helper will be keeping a fairly close eye on you in these early days. In Britain, the community midwife comes every day for at least ten days after you leave the hospital and go home. The health visitor will also pay some calls at this time. They'll want to make sure that everything is going well, and their job is to answer any questions you might have and to deal with anything which might be worrying you. For example, they're trained to help you with breastfeeding, and the midwife will also probably help you to bath the baby at least once. There are also some voluntary organisations which can help you, and you'll find some addresses at the end of the book.

One problem for many young parents can be that everybody loads them up with advice. You'll have lots of visitors, and you'll find that maiden aunts, Granny and even the postman will suddenly become transformed into sages who claim they know everything about babies. You'll need to be careful on two counts; the first is that you'll find most of the advice is contradictory, and the second is that other people can be very sensitive at such times.

Remember that becoming a grandparent can come as something of a shock, too, and that when you have a baby your own parents are going to have to make some adjustments themselves. Most new grandparents are very happy, of course, but it can also bring back all sorts of memories, and make them feel old. Obviously, your own parents *are* a good source of advice – they've been through what you're experiencing – but times change, and we all have a tendency to ignore our parents' advice at times. New dads can play a very useful role here by controlling the flow of visitors, and by making sure that everybody gets their fair share of cuddles with the baby – and also that they don't outstay their welcome. And as far as the advice is concerned – take the advice you need or like and forget the rest. If you're worried about your baby, ask your doctor's advice *first*.

Surviving – and still sane

There will come a time, whether it's at two months, six months or a year, when you'll suddenly realise that life has settled down – a little. You'll realise that you've survived, and that you're probably still almost sane. In a way it's the most dangerous time of all.

When Emma was a couple of months old she had settled down remarkably well. In particular, she began to miss out the night feeds – and sleep peacefully through the night. Life suddenly became wonderful, and both Sally and I began to think that being a parent was the easiest job in the world.

Inside a month Emma had begun a period of her life which nearly drove us both to despair. She started crying all night, every night. After a few weeks we both looked like the living dead; and we both felt as if we'd been tortured by the Spanish Inquisition continuously for several years. It was all made worse by the fact that we had had that month of peace and quiet and refreshing sleep. It was a shattering blow.

There was also something else in us which didn't help matters at all, something very simple and on the surface so good that it's hard to believe it can make the business of being a parent a nightmare. That was our enthusiasm, our desire to get everything right, our keenness. We wanted to be *perfect* parents, and as you've probably realised by now, that's the worst thing to do. If you set out trying to be perfect in anything, you're only likely to be disappointed.

Nowhere is this more true than in parenthood. Everybody – and I mean *everybody* – makes all sorts of mistakes, even doctors and midwives when it comes to having their own children. I'm not talking about serious mistakes, I'm talking about things like not putting a nappy on properly or getting those tiny fingers caught in a jumper at an awkward angle and provoking a heart rending cry. I'll never forget just how upset Sally got one day when she was cutting Emma's finger nails because she accidentally snipped some flesh at the corner of a nail and made that tiny finger bleed.

Remember that most first time parents are terribly keen, too, and of course, that's a very good thing. But it means that, like us, you'll want to change your baby's nappy every time she makes it the tiniest bit wet. With second and subsequent babies you won't love them or care for them any the less, but you'll have learned that you don't have to be so fussy all the time. Leaving your baby in her nappy until she's done enough to make it worth your while to change it will save you a lot of effort – and washing, although you still shouldn't leave her in a wet nappy *too* long because there's a chance that doing so could lead to a case of nappy rash. By that time – or even before – you may have realised that disposable nappies could save you a whole lot of washing.

But it's hard to think of all these things when everything is so new and frightening. Another thing few first time parents realise is that their babies are remarkably tough and resilient creatures, and that *they* also want to settle down, too. Some time during their first year, life will become more settled, easier, more familiar – and when that happens depends very much on your baby's development.

8. How your child develops

IN THIS CHAPTER I'm going to look at how children develop in the first few years of their lives. During that time they achieve some remarkable things. For example, at birth they can neither understand what is said to them nor reply – but by the age of five they're able to hold quite complicated conversations, and they can use language for all sorts of different purposes. At birth they're physically helpless and can't even raise their own heads; five years later they can run, jump and have made a real start on the long journey to the full independence of adulthood.

You might think that this is all very simple and straightforward. After all, you might say, aren't children designed to grow up into adults? Most of us do exactly that, don't we? We do, but it's not quite so easy as all that. In fact child development is a very complicated subject, and that's why I've devoted a whole chapter to it. Even so, I'll only be able to draw the broadest, simplest picture of how this remarkable and fascinating process unfolds.

There is one other, much more important reason for writing this chapter, though. It's quite simple – the more you know about child development, the more you'll be able to make sure that *your* child gets as close as she can to developing her full potential. In this context it's vital to keep in mind that a child doesn't grow up in isolation. She'll grow up in a family and is therefore part of a unique collection of unique individuals, all of whom influence each other enormously. The arrival of a new baby means that everybody in the family has to make adjustments and come to terms with a changed way of life. These adjustments will continue because the changes will too. A family isn't a static, unchanging structure; it's a dynamic, living, growing unit, and the main driving force of change within it in the early years is none other than the child herself. As she grows and changes, so her parents will have to react to her in new ways, which will in turn stimulate her to develop in new directions.

I used the word *potential* above, and that's very important. Each child inherits certain things from her parents, and these things aren't just physical either. We inherit all sorts of traits and talents and personality characteristics from our parents, and scientists are only just beginning to realise just how much our genes determine. Any parent knows that each child is born with a unique character which is obvious almost from the first day of life.

But how that character and those talents develop depends very much on what happens during the child's life. We know that a healthy child born to tall, fit and athletic parents has a marvellous chance of turning out the same way. But she'll only develop her full physical potential if she gets the right balance of healthy foods throughout her childhood, and is given plenty of opportunities for healthy exercise. In many ways the same is true of our emotional and intellectual potential. We can be born with a sunny disposition and the potential for real wisdom and intelligence. But we still need to be helped to make the most of them. Some people *do* overcome the problems of a deprived childhood and achieve success and happiness. But how much better it is for a child to grow up secure, happy and intellectually stimulated.

That's why it's so important for parents to know as much as they can about child development. If you have children, the development of their potential rests in your hands. You can help them to grow up fit, healthy, happy and intelligent; and to do that you need to know what to do and when to do it. Of course a lot of this is strictly common sense — but it's surprising just how often some parents ignore the obvious.

But I need to make one very important point. During the rest of this chapter I will be saying things like "most children reach this stage at six months, a year, five years of age . . ." These ages refer to averages; that is, most children do achieve these things at around the same age. However, individual children can still learn to walk, for example, very early or very late in comparison to the average and still be completely normal. In one section we'll be looking at what happens when a child is found to be a late developer or has a specific problem.

A bundle of talents

Doctors who have studied child development divide it into four main areas. These are: the *personal/social*, which includes things like how a child develops knowledge of and relationships with the people around her; *gross motor development*, which is basically how a child learns to become mobile and walk and run; *fine motor development*, which is how the child develops the use and skills of her hands; and *language*, which is how a child learns to understand and use humanity's unique means of communication.

I'm going to be looking at all these areas, but of course in reality it's virtually impossible to divide them up in this way. A child is one complete individual, and although there may be bursts of development in any one of these areas while the others seem to be fairly static, development goes on in all of them continually, throughout childhood. They overlap, too, and a breakthrough in one area – like learning to walk – will bring new opportunities in others, new areas to explore and conquer.

Let's start by looking at what a newborn baby is capable of. In Chapter 4 we looked at how a baby develops in the womb, and saw that by the end of the nine months of pregnancy the baby could hear and see and had a fairly well developed brain and nervous system. In fact that's how she arrives in the world, but once she's out of the womb, her other senses can also come into operation. It used to be thought at one time that newborn babies were practically deaf and blind, but we now know this isn't true. They can see, hear, taste, smell and feel – and they can do all of them very well indeed.

Newborn babies are a bundle of talents. Something else they can do – and which they've been practising in the womb for months – is *suck*. Obviously, this is a very important ability, and that's reflected in just how skilful newborn babies are at it. They also have what's called the *rooting reflex*. If stroked around the mouth or on the cheek, the baby will turn towards the source of the stimulation and start to suck; it's a most useful talent for someone who's going to get all her food through sucking. It's also amazing to see a baby who might only be minutes old turning to the breast in this way.

A baby is also born with a few other reflexes. There's the *startle* or *Moro* reflex, for instance. If she's startled, a newborn will fling her limbs out, then bring them back in what appears to be an 'embrace'. Another reflex can be seen when a baby is held upright in a 'standing' position. When the soles of her feet touch a surface, she appears to take a few steps – almost as if she was trying to walk. These reflexes are thought to be connected with the survival needs of our remote, primitive ancestors – perhaps helping babies to cling on to parents who were swinging through trees or otherwise very active soon after birth. Obviously they don't have much use these days, and in any case, they soon disappear – usually within a few weeks.

But they do point to the fact that a newborn baby is interested in one thing above all, and that's *survival*. Some other facts bear this out. For example, it's known that a newborn baby can focus on objects eight to fifteen inches from her face, and that's about the distance her mother's face will be from hers during a feed. It's also been discovered that newborn babies are interested above all in human faces, and that given a choice, they'll look at a face in preference to anything else. They're also interested in human voices, and there is some evidence which suggests they can even recognise their mother's voice as soon as they're born. It could well be so; after all, the baby has been listening to her mother's voice from inside the womb throughout pregnancy.

What all this adds up to, however, is a baby who is designed to respond to the people who are going to take care of her – and to make those people respond to her. I've already said that parenthood has to be learned, but certain things about it do simply come naturally. Both mothers and fathers who have been observed with their newborn babies react in very similar ways. They seek out eye contact with the baby, they cuddle her close with her head on the left hand side of their chests, in a position where the baby can hear the heart beating. They have been observed speaking in a special way to their babies; it's not exactly baby talk, but they do speak in a higher tone, and more slowly, and they repeat what they say often. As we'll see, this is just what the doctor ordered when it comes to the baby learning to use language.

All this centres in the early days and weeks on the activity which is closest to the baby's heart — feeding. When she's not feeding, the baby is likely to be in a deep, contented sleep; but when she is feeding, she really makes the most of her time awake. We also know that her 'survival kit' comes with one final, essential ingredient — she can tell the difference between sweet and bitter tastes, and infinitely prefers sweet ones. And breast milk happens to be sweet. At this time all the baby is really interested in is surviving by satisfying her needs. If you make sure she's fed, warm and cuddled, then you won't be going very far wrong. These early days are a transition period — and they're a transition for the baby as much as they are for you. She's learning to live in a big, bright and noisy world — and she can't take in too much yet.

Developing downwards

But it won't be long before she's ready to start exploring the world around. Of course she's limited by the fact that she can't get around, and to start with she can't control her eyes very well or co-ordinate them with her other senses. That's why the early months will be a period when she concentrates her efforts on gaining control of as much of her body as she can.

Her development will, in fact, proceed downwards. That's because control of her body depends on her brain and nervous system becoming more mature. As it does, she gains control of her eyes and head, then her hands and slowly the rest of her body until finally she conquers those far flung outposts, her legs and feet. She also has to develop the strength and co-ordination of muscles and groups of muscles, and all of this takes time and effort.

All this is also related to that overwhelming survival instinct and her interest in the people who are taking care of her. A newborn baby will listen to the sound of her mother's voice, but can't turn her eyes to look for her. By the age of four or five weeks, however, she'll be able to do just that. At about six weeks, she'll also begin to explore one hand with the other, and by around eight weeks, she's likely to look at her hands properly for the first time.

This is a very important moment, because it's the beginning of a very important skill indeed, and that's *hand-eye co-ordination*. We tend not to think about this skill once we acquire it, but if you look at a baby struggling to learn it you'll be amazed at your own ability to thread needles, grasp hammers or the fine handles of bone china cups, or even pick up a tiny piece of fluff from the carpet. In the early months the baby concentrates on learning how to grasp things which interest her and on bringing them to her. Most often she'll put them to her mouth to explore their texture and taste, and that's because her mouth is probably her most sensitive – and favourite – organ, as it's where that most important of all things comes to her, her food.

Of course, she'll continue to refine and improve this skill throughout her childhood. But to keep up the pace of development, she'll need to be able to do more than just lie on her back. That's why at about the same time as she begins to use her hands, she'll probably start to raise her head and gain more control of its movements. By the age of two months, many babies can raise their heads for a while when they're placed on their stomach. A couple of months later, she'll probably be able to hold her head up and look around if she's helped into a sitting position. When she's six to eight months old she's likely to be able to sit herself up.

By the time she's got this far, your baby will be well on the way to learning to walk. She will have been helping this process along for a few months by playing with her feet and legs, which is something all babies seem to love doing.

The next stage for most babies is pulling themselves up from sitting to standing. They'll use anything which is handy for this – the furniture, toys, their parents – and they'll spend a lot of time falling back on their bottoms. Most babies start doing this between the ages of eight and ten months. At about the same time, many babies start to crawl, although some miss out this stage entirely, while others shuffle along on their bottoms instead. Crawling on all fours takes some mastering, and many babies are delighted when they can do it. For the first time in their lives they achieve real mobility and it opens up whole new worlds for them.

Within a few months they'll be progressing from crawling to standing and taking a few unaided steps. This usually happens some time between twelve and fifteen months, and they'll be very unsteady at first, with lots of wobbling and tumbles over all sorts of enormous obstacles like the edge of the carpet. But once your baby's taken her first steps, she'll hardly look back. It's not the end of her gross motor development by any means – she's still got the delights of running, jumping and climbing to discover – but it does mark the end of the beginning.

The name of the game

Remember that all this gross motor development isn't happening in isolation. You'll be helping her all the time, and during that first fifteen months in which your baby learns to walk, you'll also have built a very complex relationship with her and a large part of that will be based on language.

Some experts now believe that human babies are born with an instinctive ability and desire to learn to speak. Whether or not this is true – and I for one think it's pretty obvious – there's no doubt that our babies are surrounded by language from the time they're born. We talk to them as we rock and cuddle them, right from the beginning. We sing nursery rhymes and songs to them to try and get them to go to sleep. We talk and talk and talk to them all the time.

All this communication isn't one way, though. It's been discovered, in fact, that our babies tend to lead and we follow. Close studies of babies and their parents have shown that if your baby sticks out her tongue, you're likely to imitate her. If she starts making a noise – whether it's a gurgle, a whoop or a giggle – you're likely to imitate that too. What you're doing is teaching your baby that you can do anything she can. You're teaching her that we can make noises when we want to and that we can *communicate*.

All this early communication is vital, even though most of the time we're doing it unconsciously. A pattern of mutual response develops as your baby grows older and more mature, and it works through everything that both of you do – gestures, expressions, movements, sounds, tones of voice and the rhythm of what you're saying. Rhythm is very important. We tend to talk to our babies instinctively in a high-pitched, musical, rhythmical and repetitive way. This makes it easier and more attractive for them to follow our voices, and it also usually includes lots of laughing and smiling. All this is vital; and soon your baby will be babbling back at you during these conversations as much as she can.

Again, it's a question of learning to control the complex muscles and groups of muscles which operate the physical apparatus we use when we speak – our mouths, tongues, lips, voice box and so on. Babies babble away, imitating what they hear around them, gaining more and more control over the means to communicate. They practise a lot, just as you do when you're learning a foreign language; and it's all Greek to them to begin with!

At any rate, your baby will pass through a stage some time in the second half of her first year, or the beginning of her second year, when what she's babbling away in sounds almost like real language. Eventually she'll say her first recognisable word, an event which can occur at any time between the ages of nine and eighteen months. Some children suddenly explode into language, while others seem to pick it up very slowly, almost at the rate of one word a week. Whatever pace they go at, their first words are bound to be about the people and things which are important to them – 'dadda', 'mumma' and so on. As far as late talking is concerned, there does seem to be a difference between the sexes in this respect, with boys often beginning to talk later than girls. There's nothing abnormal about this though.

That first word – like the first few steps – isn't an end in itself, but a beginning. During the second and third years of a child's life she makes enormous strides in language, and she'll continue to develop linguistically long after that. She will, that is, so long as she continues to get the sort of stimulation we've been talking about in this section. It's a simple fact, proved by research studies, that if you don't talk to your child, she won't talk back. Of course, the opposite is also true; the more you talk to your child, the more language of all sorts that she's exposed to and the more fun it all is, the quicker and better she'll develop her language abilities.

In this context it's very much up to you. Take the use of books, for example. There are an enormous number of children's books around today, and very many of them are of a high standard, in terms of both story and pictures. Publishers are also increasingly producing books aimed at very young children and babies. It's been shown that children who have more books read to them from an early age learn to speak more quickly, have wider vocabularies and find it easier to learn to read when they get to school. So it's up to you – if you make it your business to expose your children to books, you'll be doing them a real service.

Stimulation is the name of the game. The more stimulation of all sorts that your child gets, the better. New experiences stimulate the brain to develop, and the more mature the brain and nervous system become, the more experiences your child becomes capable of appreciating. Given the chance, most normal children will soak up everything that's offered to them – books, television, music, songs, nursery rhymes. They'll enjoy everything, and if the experiences come wrapped in fun (which many childhood experiences do, you've only got to think of nursery rhymes to understand that) so much the better.

One point which I think it's very important to make is that when it comes to looking after children, there should be no difference between mothers and fathers. Men are just as capable of being good 'mothers' as women. Children don't mind whether they're being looked after full time by a man or a woman; all that matters to them is that they get the right sort of care and stimulation.

In broad terms, there is no inborn difference between men and women when it comes to parenthood; the only differences are the ones I talked about in Chapter 2, the ones which are drummed into you as you grow up. And it's up to you to make sure that your children don't suffer the sort of pressure I talked about there. You can give your sons dolls to play with, and help them to understand that it's not 'sissy' to do so. You can get a first-born son to help you with his baby brother or sister. You can encourage your daughters to be independent, to think of themselves as potential career women and not just simply as somebody's eventual wife or mother.

It's vital to think of these things from early on because there's evidence that the differences between boys and girls which I've talked about start to develop at a very young age. The pressures on us all to conform to the standard male and female stereotypes are enormous and very, very subtle, and it's only by a conscious effort to break the mould that you can help your children to live different, fuller lives. If Dad does the washing up, puts the kids to bed and takes a large part in bringing up the children, his sons will see that as a normal part of life. And if Mum is independent, with interests and perhaps a career of her own as well as a family, then her daughters will have more of an example to follow. But it's important to keep in mind that your children's attitude to society and their own futures begins here and now, in their babyhood and childhood.

Learning through play

That, of course, brings us to the subject of play, which is, I suppose, the word we most commonly associate with childhood. Play is, quite simply, a child's way of learning about the world. We tend to think of play as being very unimportant, trivial even; but for a child it's one of the most important, valuable things of all.

For a long time, a baby's most valuable playthings are his parents. They do all sorts of wonderful, fascinating things, and the baby will want more and more contact with them as she gets older. Those 'conversations' in the process of learning to talk are play; you supply your baby with the raw material which she absorbs and experiments with in all sorts of creative ways.

There are several different types of play, all of which are important. First of all there's *physical play*, the running, jumping sort of play that all children indulge in once they become more mobile. Then there's a finer sort of physical play which we'll call *hand play*, and which involves using the hands in different ways. Then there's *role-playing*, which becomes very important. This covers all those 'going shopping' games, and playing 'postmen' or 'doctors and nurses'. Linked with this is *social play* – the sort of play which involves playing together with other children co-operatively.

The first two types of physical play have a very important role to fill in a child's development. When a four-month-old baby lies in her cot and kicks her legs in the air she's playing with a real, if unconscious, purpose – and that's to help her physical development forward. Similarly, when a baby plays with a rattle or explores a soft toy with her hands she's developing those vital hand-eye skills which will serve her throughout her life.

Obviously, these types of play continue to be important throughout childhood. If you've ever looked at a collection of two, three, four or five-year-olds at a nursery school, kindergarten or school, you'll have noticed that they seem to be in constant motion. They run everywhere while they're playing; they use their hands constantly, picking up and exploring everything which comes their way. Over the years they become better and better at running, jumping, climbing and using their hands. Some are faster than others, stronger, more athletic, and these talents will become apparent as they grow up. But every child loves physical activity, and the more they get, the better. Healthy, enjoyable exercise at this stage of life lays the foundations for a healthy body in adulthood.

Role-playing builds on the imitation which we've already seen at work in those 'conversations' between parent and baby in the early months. During the second and third years of a child's life, she'll become increasingly fascinated by all the things that go on around her, and she'll start to imitate them. She'll imitate you cooking the breakfast and making the beds. She'll imitate the postman delivering the letters and the bus driver driving the bus. She'll spend hours in long drawn out games of going to the shops, going on holiday, visiting Grandma and so on.

All this imitation is the sincerest form of flattery as far as your child is concerned. She's so interested in what's going on around her that she wants to absorb it and play a part in it. She imitates so that she can understand, and also because – like all human beings – she's creative and she wants to build new games, new structures, out of the experiences she has, the things and people which surround her. It's how she learns about the world and its ways, and this role-playing will go on for years.

Social play is linked to it because you need help with a lot of these games. What good is a doctor without a patient, for example, or a bus driver without a passenger? Children need to play with other children to make these sort of games really worthwhile: But there's another reason to promote social play; it helps your child to learn how to get on with other people. Very few of us live the lives of hermits, and so we need to develop the skills necessary to live and work with other people. Of course children learn this sort of thing through the family, but as they grow older they need contact with 'outsiders'. Playschools, nursery schools or kindergarten later play an important part in this context, but just simple visits to friends who have children can provide the right sort of contact – and give the parents some welcome personal relaxation and reassurance as well.

Talking of play brings the subject of toys to mind. The two naturally go together, as I well know; I find it a continual source of amazement that three small children can accumulate as many toys as mine have. Of course, doting grandparents, uncles and aunts are mostly to blame, and it's good for children to have lots of toys. But it's also important to remember certain things as far as toys are concerned.

First, you should always make sure that a toy bought for any child is *safe*. These days in most countries there are fairly strict regulations about toy safety. These say that toys should be made of safe, non-toxic materials and that they shouldn't have sharp edges, pinch points or small parts which could be pulled off and which a baby or child could choke on. Major toy companies work very hard at making sure their toys conform to the regulations, but it's always worth checking. There are still occasional cases of children being harmed by soft toys stuffed with poisonous materials or cutting themselves on toys which are badly designed. If you're ever in doubt about a particular toy, don't buy it – or get rid of it if it comes as a present.

Secondly, it's important to make sure that your child gets the right toys at the right age. For example, it's no good buying a complicated computer toy for a small baby, or a giant doll for a toddler. They just won't get any play value from them. Babies need bright, colourful toys which make noises and stimulate them; toys like rattles, cuddly animals; toys which play tunes and ring or rattle. Toddlers need toys to pull along and walk with, and older children need toys which will stimulate their minds in role-playing and social play. Throughout childhood children need toys for outside physical play, like hoops and bouncing balls, bikes and trikes and trolleys and buckets and spades – the right sizes for the right age. Most parents find that their children let them know what sorts of toys they want – whether they can afford them is another matter!

Thirdly, every Christmas you'll hear someone saying that children always play with the wrapping their presents come in more than the expensive presents themselves. That old cliché hides a real truth – you *don't* need to spend a fortune on toys for your children. It's nice if you've got the money and can afford to do so, but few young families have much spare cash at all, and many parents feel guilty because they can't buy their children all the toys they want – or as many as the children next door have got.

My children have plenty of toys, but some of their favourite games involve things which didn't really cost anything at all. When Helen was small she would spend hours playing with some saucepans and a ladle – sometimes she would be 'cooking the dinner', and sometimes she'd be playing the bass drum in a parade! We've also got an old bin full of cast-off clothes which goes under the name of the 'dressing up box'. My children can find whole costumes in there, and they spend hours dressing up and going on long 'shopping trips' from room to room. We've built 'houses' out of old cardboard packing cases, and a cheap old paddling pool in the garden in the summer probably gives them all more fun than anything else they've got.

And when they have to spend time indoors, they've got pencils, paper and paints, crayons, old egg boxes and cartons to cut up, sellotape and masking tape and glue; our walls are plastered with 'sculptures', 'models' and paintings which I think knock Picasso's daubs into a cocked hat. All these things play an essential part in their development, too; holding paintbrushes and crayons helps a child develop the vital skills she's going to need when she learns to write. I've watched my children spend whole days doing things like that, and they do them with great concentration, interest and application. They're enjoying themselves – and their enjoyment helps them develop all the skills they're going to build on when they get to school.

Living with a child

You may have realised by now that all this play and stimulation will involve you as parents a great deal. It can't be any other way, of course; you're the only people who can supply the toys and the stimulation, and you're the only people who are around all the time. A parent is a child's favourite plaything, and that stays true for many years during childhood.

Once a baby gets past the eating-sleeping-feeding stage, she'll be ever more ready for stimulation. She'll demand it in fact, and she'll want to play all the time. The problems come because you can't devote every waking minute to entertaining your child, however much you'd like to. Meals have to be cooked, housework done, shops visited, other people (like your partner) talked to and so on. It can be very frustrating for both parent and child when they begin to realise that life has to be organised and lived, and that all that warm, stimulating contact often comes a fairly long way down the list of priorities.

Guilt can creep in here, too, especially when you read books like this which tell you that your child needs all the stimulation she can get to make sure she develops her full potential. The thing to remember is that very often it's not so much the *quantity* of the stimulation your child gets which matters, but the *quality*. It's far better to spend ten minutes playing in an enjoyable way than half an hour with your mind on other things. Besides which, many parents soon learn to turn everything into a game. You'll find that you'll probably become an expert at keeping up a running commentary on what you're doing while you're doing it; you'll point out everything of interest on the way to the shops; you'll find yourself singing nursery rhymes at the top of your voice in the oddest of places – like the supermarket.

You'll also find yourself losing your temper, and at times feeling that you simply don't want to play another game or read another children's book. That's because you'll be tired and under pressure, like all parents. For each new stage in your child's development can make life busier and more complicated.

For example, once your child becomes mobile it means she'll be able to follow you around – and she will. She'll also be into everything; she'll climb on the furniture, pull things off shelves, fall over and hurt herself, pull the cat's tail and generally make your life a nightmare. It's at this stage that you have to make sure that where you live is as safe and baby-proof as possible, otherwise she could do herself some real damage.

But the problems aren't simply ones of safety and mobility. By the time your child gets into her second year she will already have shown definite signs of an independent will – she'll be *misbehaving*. This is a very difficult area, because what one person thinks of as bad behaviour another would put down to high spirits or playfulness. But there's no doubt that bad behaviour is one of the most crucial areas of child development, and it's all linked with the development of the relationship between parents and child.

The first thing to keep in mind about young children is that they tend to see everything from one point of view – their own – and in black and white terms. In short, they're supreme egotists who want everything their own way. It's hardly surprising, since their survival in the early months is based on egotism – they have to make sure their need for food and warmth is satisfied, and nothing else matters to them. It takes time to learn that they can't have everything they want immediately, and that sometimes they can't have some things at all. Children also have very little patience; it's no good saying to a demanding two-year-old that you'll read her a story later – all she knows is that she wants it *now* and you're not giving it to her.

It isn't until later on that children begin to operate on the principle of give and take, and learn how to wait their turn, wait for what they want, and generally pick up the social skills we adults prize so much. In the early months and years their reactions to being thwarted are often direct and very negative. They shout. They scream. They throw colossal tantrums. They kick out, bite, pinch, bash their heads against walls, throw things, smash their favourite toys and make themselves positively unpleasant. Some children even hold their breath until they go blue in the face, terrifying their poor parents.

When you first begin to see all these things happening before your very eyes, when you realise that the sweet, lovable little baby you brought into the world is capable of such appalling behaviour, you can be very shocked indeed. It's all completely normal, though. One of the most important lessons anyone learns in life is that you can't possibly have your own way all of the time. At the age of two or three a child begins to learn exactly that.

It's a very harsh lesson for most children to learn, and it's important for parents to make it as easy for them as they can. There isn't a lot you can do about the tantrums and the bad behaviour. There isn't much you can do about the fact that you'll react strongly to your children's bad behaviour at times, too. Indeed, if you throw a tantrum, in return, once in a while – as most parents do – your children will realise that everybody, even adults, have their limits, and can lose their tempers, a very important piece of learning.

But you can keep in mind that staying cool will make your children's bad behaviour a lot easier to deal with. It's also important to remember that much so-called bad behaviour is in fact the result of a child's immaturity. A two-year-old doesn't knock over her drink on purpose very often – it's more likely to be an accident. Many tantrums are also the result of sheer frustration when she can't achieve something she wants to. You'll soon get to know the difference, though – and work out what steps to take accordingly.

A lot of the worst bad behaviour is the result of arguments and fighting between children, especially brothers and sisters. Children can be very unpleasant to each other, whether they're related or not. Of course, this is all part of learning to live with other people. On a very basic level, you find out that if you pull someone's hair then she's likely to do the same thing to you – and that your parents won't like it very much!

That brings us to the subject of *discipline*, one of the knottiest problems any parent has to face. Some parents believe in *physical punishment*, and smack their children when they're naughty. Others don't, and use other methods to get their children to behave themselves. Physical punishment can be a problem in certain cases, although there's no doubt that many parents do still use smacking as their main method of discipline.

I'll be looking at the question of smacking in more detail in the next chapter. But it's important to say that children *need* limits of some sort in their lives, they need to know that sometimes they can only go so far. It is, after all, the only way they can learn many things about themselves, the world and the people around them. Limits also give them the security of knowing that you care and that you're looking after them. When you tell your child off you're actually helping her – although it's sometimes hard to believe.

Before we leave the subject of bad behaviour, it's important to remember one more thing. Children at any age can be lovely. Tearaway toddlers can suddenly transform themselves into little angels; the child who you could have happily strangled ten minutes ago, now creeps up behind you to kiss you, unasked, on the back of the neck.

In fact, as they grow older, my children give me more and more pleasure. Very often I love being with them. They're fun, they're stimulating, they're interesting, they're wonderful to be with, they make me laugh. All this not only makes up for the times when they're fighting or screaming, it's also quite simply good in itself. I know that if I didn't have children, my life would not be as rich or as full of opportunities for love and enjoyment; and also that the nicer I am to my children, the nicer they are to me – usually. It's very important for you to realise that these benefits are a real advantage when it comes to becoming a parent; they make it worth all the bother.

Still dependent

You'll certainly be looking after your children for many years to come, in every way. For example, a child will still be in nappies long after she's learned to walk, and that's because it takes her longer to learn to control her bladder and bowels than it does her legs. That means you'll be changing nappies – and therefore being up to your elbows in their contents – when your child is two, three and perhaps even older.

Toilet training their children is something all parents have to face, and it can cause a lot of anxiety. The simple fact is that it can take a lot of patience, but most children achieve complete control of their bladders and bowels before they go to school. The key is to take a child out of nappies and start using a pot or toilet seat when *she* is ready – trying to force the pace will only lead to problems. It's also important not to become anxious about a child who seems to be taking a long time over becoming toilet trained – she'll only pick up your anxiety, and feel anxious about it herself. That will only help to make the whole process take longer.

Most children are out of nappies in the day long before they're dry at night. One in ten five-year-olds still wets the bed, and bedwetting is a problem which can last for years in a minority of children. Even those children who achieve control without any problems often have accidents in the day or the night. It's important to treat these for what they are – minor setbacks on the road to independence – rather than 'punish' a child for something she probably would have avoided if she'd been able to.

Something else you're going to have to do is to introduce your baby to solid food. It's called weaning, and most parents do this when their babies are between the ages of three and six months. It's not usually a good idea to start them on solids before that, as there's a chance they might become allergic to certain foods, something which can lead to all sorts of problems. Small babies don't have teeth, so at first they can only cope with mushed up foods which have about the same consistency as milk.

Their teeth start to come at about the age of six months – although again, this can happen earlier or later – and most children have a complete set of their first or *milk teeth* by the time they're two and a half. This process is called *teething*, and it means that your child will gradually be able to cope with more types of food which involve chewing. It is, naturally enough, vital to keep two things in mind when you're preparing food for a small child – its quantity and quality.

Small children can very quickly become overweight if they eat too many sweet, sticky foods, lots of cakes, sweets, white bread and so on. Children eat what they like – and they'll eat tons of this sort of food if they can get away with it. That's why it's important for you to make sure they eat a balanced, natural diet.

That isn't the only sort of problem your children's eating habits can bring. Most children soon discover that being fussy over their food, generally misbehaving at meal times or simply refusing to eat are all marvellous ways of getting a rise out of their parents. You will find yourself worrying about whether your child eats enough, and this sort of behaviour can be a real problem with most children at some stage. It's vital to remember that no very young child is capable of starving herself to death, although some seem determined to – and also that by allowing your child to see she can get at you in this way you'll only prolong the problem. Stay cool – however hard it may be – and eventually the problem will sort itself out. In general, a healthy child who gets plenty of healthy exercise will have a healthy appetite.

Your child will also be dependent on you in other ways. Few children are capable of dressing themselves properly much before the age of five, and that means every morning you'll have to spend time washing, combing and dressing a small child. That can be a very difficult task, especially when the child in question is feeling difficult and unco-operative.

Mornings make me think of sleep, a subject never far from any parent's mind. I mentioned that your baby will probably start sleeping through the night at some time early in her first year, and that life will then become a little easier. The harsh fact which I neglected to mention was that once you become a parent, sleep will never be the same again. Most parents of babies find that even though they're not taking night feeds, they still wake up from time to time. Some unlucky parents even find that they have a baby who apparently doesn't want to sleep at all.

I know we went through a very bad patch with Emma. From about the age of three months onwards, every night she woke and refused to be comforted. She screamed as we rocked her, she screamed when we put her in her cot, she screamed and screamed and screamed. After a few weeks of this we were at the end of our tether. She eventually got over it, but even now at the age of five she still sometimes wakes in the middle of the night because of a nightmare, and may need comforting. I know many, many parents who have had the same experience – and worse ones – and the simple fact is that if you've got children, you have to expect to be 'on call' in the middle of the night throughout most of their childhood.

We solved our particular problem by taking Emma into bed with us, something which we had been reluctant to do. It worked almost immediately, and made us realise that all Emma had wanted was some security and cuddles. Instead, for a long time, we had simply offered her anxiety, fatigue and bad temper – no wonder she cried! Many parents, however, don't like the idea of sharing their bed with their children, and it has to be said that once your child gets into the habit of sleeping with you, it's very hard to get her out of it. Emma now sleeps in her own bed, thank heavens, but Helen still wakes up every night and comes into ours. I don't mind most of the time, but it can sometimes be a little disconcerting to wake up with your daughter's foot in your eye. Many parents start out saying they'll never have their children in bed with them – and end up succumbing simply to get a better night's sleep. Obviously, as your child grows older, she'll be less prone to night wandering and waking you up – but it's something which can last for a long time.

Your child and the doctor

Your child will be, therefore, dependent on you for almost every aspect of her life. She's physically dependent on you; dependent on you, in many ways, for her intellectual development, at least until she starts school; she's dependent on you for her security, and for her emotional well-being. She's very dependent on you for that most important ingredient of all human relationships, some would even say of all human life – love.

She's also dependent on you for her health. You can take positive steps to ensure your child is developing normally and is healthy. In most countries parents are encouraged to take their babies and children along to the doctor for regular developmental and health checks.

In Britain, for example, parents are given appointments to take their children to a *well baby clinic*. The main point of these clinics is simply to make sure that your baby is healthy and stays so. You'll be able to talk to a health visitor or doctor about any problems you might have, and they'll be glad to give you advice about any area of your child's development or family life. Their other main purpose is to make sure that your child is developing normally. The doctor will probably want to see your child at regular intervals and give her tests especially designed to do this – at the ages of six weeks, six to eight months, one year, eighteen months, two or three years and then just before she starts school.

These regular checks will make sure that if there is a problem, it will be detected as early as possible. The sooner any developmental problem or illness is discovered, the sooner the correct treatment can be applied. That generally means a child has a better chance of overcoming the problem – or learning to live with it at the very least.

There are many different types of problems which are detected in these checks. For example, it might be found that a child who is slow in learning to talk is actually wholly or partially deaf. Some children who are slow in developing in general may be found to have some sort of brain damage. As with premature babies and threatened miscarriages, doctors are continually pushing back the boundaries of how much children like these can be helped. Treatment for the deaf ranges – depending on what the cause of the deafness is – from surgery to speech therapy, and they can be helped in many ways. The same is true of most of the problems detected at the clinic, which shows just how important it is for you to take your child along to every appointment. In this sense, these check-ups are just as important as the antenatal check-ups you have during pregnancy.

Children are also usually immunised against various illnesses at the clinic. This is a means of making you immune to a disease by exposing you to a small, carefully prepared dose of it. It's a technique with which we're all familiar, and one which we tend to take for granted; but it's been instrumental in making dangerous diseases like diphtheria, tetanus, polio and tuberculosis virtually a thing of the past, at least in the developed countries.

In recent years there's been a lot of publicity about the risks of *whooping cough immunisation*. The facts are simple. Whooping cough is a very dangerous and unpleasant disease which can cause a child great suffering, and sometimes kills. However, a very few children react badly to the vaccine and even suffer brain damage. It's important to get the facts clear in your mind, though – this happens to very, very few children, and there are certain things which doctors know put certain children at risk. One of these is a family history of convulsions or fits. It's also vital that as many children as possible should be protected against this disease; scares about brain damage which led many parents not to have their children immunised also caused whooping cough epidemics. If your child is at risk, then your doctor won't give her the vaccine – but if she isn't, she should have it. If you're in any doubt at all, it's something you should talk over with your doctor.

Even if you do take your child to the clinic regularly, she's still bound to suffer from various illnesses from time to time. Children catch all sorts of coughs, colds and infections, and that's because they're not immune to the bacteria and viruses which surround us throughout our lives. In fact we pick up immunity to the common illnesses – like many of the viruses which cause colds, measles, chickenpox and so on – by having them as children.

That doesn't make them any easier to deal with, and one of the most distressing experiences for any parent is to sit and watch her child racked with any illness, however mild. It can be quite terrifying to realise that your tiny baby has got a cold – you sometimes feel absolutely helpless and worried out of your mind. You'll also find that a sick child can be very difficult to manage; a child who feels ill is likely to be more clingy than usual, and want far more attention. It's understandable, after all – very often they don't really understand what's happening to them. I remember when Emma once had earache, she kept saying one thing to me, over and over again: "Make it go away, Daddy, make it go away . . ." I would have given anything to have made it go away then and there. I felt as if I'd failed her.

You become more accustomed to this sort of thing as your children grow older and you have more experience of it, just as you get more experience of dealing with all sorts of cuts and bruises and lumps and bumps your children collect in falls and accidents. But the worry, the deep-rooted fear for your child's health and safety, never goes away. You'll always get that churning sensation of panic when they're ill, or when they fall over, however good you become at controlling it and taking the right action. I know that whenever Emma, Helen or Thomas gets a cough or cold there's still that nagging worry about them behind my apparently cool exterior. My mother tells me that she still worries about me even now – and I'm 30!

Of course, the right action to take if you're ever worried about your child's health is to ask your doctor's advice. That doesn't mean you have to rush off to the doctor every time your baby gets the snuffles, but it's important to remember that it's always better to be safe than sorry. Most doctors will be willing to give advice over the telephone or see a baby who's under the weather. With most illnesses it's usually a question of simply looking after the baby until she gets better. Babies are remarkably tough and resilient.

So most babies grow up to be normal and healthy, and you're likely to survive their childhood, too. But there's often a cost to be paid – and that's what we'll be looking at in the next chapter.

9. Surviving parenthood

BY NOW you've got a very good idea of what it's like to become a parent. You know something about conception and pregnancy, about birth and how children develop. You know a little bit about society and its attitudes towards the whole process. In fact, you probably know a lot more about it all than either Sally or I did when it actually happened to us.

But you will also have realised that there's a lot more to it. I have talked about society and the way children of different sexes are conditioned into traditional ways of thinking. What I haven't done yet is talked about the wider issues involved; issues like work, and how society can be changed to make life more satisfying for mothers, fathers and their children. For, make no mistake about it, in the end, the main problem for most families is that society – in many countries at least – simply isn't geared to their needs.

I'm going to start this chapter by looking at the experience of young mothers who give up work to stay at home and look after their babies. Many young women are choosing a different path by going back to work after the birth. This has its own problems, as do the other ways of arranging life with children which we'll also be looking at. But there are still very many young families where the mother stays at home and the father goes out to work, and this type of family can have problems.

It seems ideal though, doesn't it? Dad the breadwinner, out there conquering the world, bringing home the bacon, ever striving in his career to give his family a better standard of living; and behind him, the 'little woman', mother and home-maker, at home with the babies, washing, cleaning, ironing, cooking. At least it seems ideal if you're of a traditional cast of mind, and however loudly some of us might protest, it seems to me that society *is* still very traditional underneath a thin veneer of 'liberation'.

It has to be said that the idea of being a full-time mother at home is still very attractive to many girls, because of the sort of conditioning they have had. It isn't all conditioning, though. Some girls find that the world of work can be very dull and boring, especially if they find themselves in underpaid, repetitive jobs with little future. It's a sad reflection on our society that many girls do find themselves in exactly that position, and in that case, it's understandable that they should see parenthood as a more stimulating and rewarding career. Of course it can well be just that, and if you decide to go into it in the positive way I've been talking about in this book, so much the better.

Again, many young women are forced out of financial necessity to return to work long before they want to. It's thought that as many as 50 per cent of mothers in the U.K. with children under five do some form of paid work, full or part-time. Many of those are doing it unwillingly, and if finances permitted, they would be only too happy to stay at home to do the demanding and rewarding job of being a full-time parent.

Other influences have a role to play, as well. I have said a lot about the need to stimulate your child, and there's a whole school of thought in child development which says that it's vital for a child to have her mother at home with her in the early, formative years. Some developmental psychologists in the past even went so far as to say that no one else will do – not even the child's father. This sort of thing connects with the strong feeling that most of us have about the link between mother and child. Most of us are, after all, the products of a society in which Dad goes out to work and Mum stays at home – so we naturally tend to follow the same path.

The crunch comes, however, when Dad actually does go back to work after the birth and leaves Mum at home with a young baby. I remember it was a very difficult moment for both Sally and me when it came. I had had a fortnight off work – as paid holiday, *not* as paternity leave – and the day came when I had to go back. Two weeks simply hadn't been enough time for us to sort ourselves out. I can recall the feeling I had as I trudged off towards the station on that bright, sunny, June

Monday morning – I felt as if I was deserting Sally in her hour of need, and it was worse because I couldn't do anything about it. I had to go back to work for that most compelling reason of all – we needed the money.

Few young mothers feel that they are being deserted when their partners go back to work; but most of them feel nervous, to say the least. For that's the moment when they're really on their own with the baby for the very first time. It seems amazing, doesn't it, after all that I've said so far, that young mothers should be left alone with their babies all day only two to three weeks after the birth. But it happens.

Two worlds

You're probably wondering why I've emphasised the isolation of young mothers. Surely there are other people around who can help? What about a young mum's friends, her relatives, the neighbours? Won't they step in to fill the breach when her partner goes back to work?

The problem is that those friends and relatives might not be around during the day either. Most young mothers work before they have children, and their friends are therefore likely to be people with jobs, too. A young mother is also unlikely to have her own parents constantly available – they're probably at work, too. In fact, she may even be living many miles away from her parents; people in our society are much more mobile than they were, and many families move great distances for a variety of reasons, the chief among them often being work. So a young mother may not have access to the network of relatives – mother, grandmother, sisters, aunts and so on – which supported previous generations.

That increased mobility has also meant the break-up of formerly close-knit neighbourhoods. Many people today – especially in cities – don't even know their neighbours, and certainly don't have much to do with them. A young mother who has just given up work will certainly not know much about her stay-at-home neighbours, and that will only serve to make her even more isolated.

What I'm talking about is something which few people even

take any notice of until they find themselves on the wrong side of it; and that's the great divide between the two worlds of modern society, work and home. Young mothers who give up work to stay at home are not just experiencing one transition, that of becoming a parent, they're also entering a world most of them haven't been in since before they went to school. There's no doubt about it; the two worlds are very different, and it's often difficult for the two to communicate with each other.

I want to concentrate here on how you're likely to feel if you find yourself in the position I've described – at home, alone during the days, looking after your baby. You'll realise from all that I've said before that you'll be feeling tired, anxious and under stress anyway as a new parent. As your partner goes out of the door and back to work, you'll also probably feel very isolated.

"I felt more lonely than I'd ever felt before," said one mother of this time. "And what made it worse was that it was so difficult to get out of the house." That's a very common experience. An apparently simple trip to the shops can end up seeming more complicated than climbing Mount Everest by the time you've got the baby fed, changed and dressed and the pram sorted out. "I never seemed to be able to get out of the house before midday when the baby was very young," one woman said to me. "It took me all morning to get everything ready."

This sort of thing can be worse in the winter, and many young mothers worry a lot about taking their babies out in the wind, rain and snow; so long as they're wrapped up warmly, a little cold weather shouldn't do them any harm. But shopping expeditions with a young baby are a key factor in your education as a young parent. You begin to realise that life is going to be more difficult on a simple, practical level, and also that society isn't going to be much help at all.

Part of it has nothing to do with society, of course; having a baby means that you've got to take her with you everywhere you go, and that means simple things like getting on a bus or train are now going to be very hard – and sometimes impossible. If you buy a large pram or baby carriage, for example, you simply won't be able to get on to any form of public transport without lots of help. That means, to all intents and purpose, unless you've got a car, that you'll be restricted in movement to as far as you can walk – which these days doesn't count as very far at all in a society geared to cars.

But society doesn't take much notice of young mothers and their babies either. You'll find out very quickly that the baby goods or baby toiletries departments are certain to be on the second floor of any supermarket or store, and that there is no easy way for a mother and baby to get up there. I'm constantly amazed at just how little thought is given to this sort of thing by the designers of shop interiors, architects and planners of shopping centres. It's only when you have to push a pram or pushchair around one of our modern cities that you realise just what an obstacle course it is for young parents and their children.

"I didn't mind that so much," said one mother. "You get used to it after a while, and as you get more experienced you even begin to learn how to cope with it a little better. What upset me more, though, was people's attitudes."

This is a very important point, and one many young mothers have mentioned to me. It's also something which few of them thought about until they came into contact with it. It relates to the point I made earlier, about other people not treating you as if you were a person in your own right, but just a mother or father. "I just felt like a second class citizen all the time," said one young mother. "It was as if I didn't matter any more."

This sort of attitude is evident in many things, not least the sort of bad design I've just talked about. In my experience, too, few people offer to help young mothers burdened with shopping and struggling to get in or out of a door designed for people without prams – and even fewer will offer help to a young father in the same position. Simply walking down the street pushing your pram can be a nightmare, as people barge into you. Modern life runs at a fast pace, and that's something you can't do when you've got a baby to look after. Of course it isn't always like that – some people are helpful, and going out with your baby can be a pleasant experience. But most parents would say that it's difficult more often than not.

The result is that many young mothers spend a lot of time at home with their babies. They do all the things that 'housewives' are supposed to do, like the washing and ironing, cleaning the house and looking after the baby. The problem with all that is very simple indeed – it's boring and repetitive. Many girls find that they're practically screaming with boredom very soon, especially if they've just given up interesting jobs. A baby is likely to keep you busy, but much of the work you'll have to do will simply be very boring, and even the most boisterous and lively baby still sleeps quite a lot – allowing you to get on with something like the washing up or the ironing.

"I thought that once I was at home on my own with the baby I'd take up some sort of hobby or do a home study course," one woman said to me. "But I never had the time or the energy. OK, maybe there were times when the baby was asleep – but there was always something to do, and it was usually something incredibly dull."

Of course, it isn't always like this. For many young mothers, the early days of parenthood are full of rewards. There's the simple fun of having a baby, and make no mistake, babies can be very enjoyable; they can also be fascinating little creatures simply to observe. You'll probably find yourself spending a lot of time admiring your baby's perfection, and marvelling at each new stage of development she reaches. You may bore other people with your tales of how she's learning to crawl, walk and talk, but you'll keep yourself happy.

Mothers at home also sometimes enjoy the freedom from going out to work that it involves. You don't have to be out and going to work in the cold and damp of winter any more; no more waiting for buses or trains, either. You can, to a large extent, plan your day how you want, although most women find that as their children get older life becomes fuller and fuller, until it can become very crowded indeed. Some women also find that having a baby and looking after a household makes them feel more competent and mature, especially if they feel that they're making a success of it.

Isolated and depressed

However, it has to be said that many young mothers do find themselves stuck indoors, alone and lonely and depressed for most of the day. However much you love the child you bring into the world, it has to be remembered that the early months can be a very difficult time for a mother at home.

I have talked about the 'baby blues' and I have said that depression can be a serious problem for young mothers. In fact, as you'll understand by now, there can be few mothers who escape depression entirely in the first year of their babies' lives. Estimates vary, but it's said that as many as one third of mothers suffer from a depression severe enough to need some help from their doctors – and many more spend a lot of time being fed up.

Depression is in fact one of the most common illnesses in the Western world, although few people even think of it as an illness. It is, and it's thought that millions of people all over the world suffer from it to one extent or another. Of course, we all have experience of feeling low, or 'down' or depressed. But depression in this sense is something which can actually affect a person's ability to live his or her life properly.

Depression as an illness can be detected by various *symptoms* – these are the signs doctors check for when trying to determine what sort of illness a person is suffering from. People who are this depressed often feel as if they'll never be happy again; they may be unable to sleep at night and have all sorts of odd aches and pains. They'll probably feel lethargic all the time, and hopeless, too. In its extreme form, depression can lead to suicide.

The figures show fairly clearly that women are more at risk from this type of depression than men, and also that young mothers of small babies at home are very much at risk. About one in 200 also suffer from a far more serious form of postnatal depression which may lead to a spell in a psychiatric hospital, and will certainly involve an extended period of medical care and treatment.

Women who suffer from this form of postnatal depression may reject their babies, and not even acknowledge that they've had them. They are likely to act in ways which we associate with the mentally ill; for example, they may have hallucinations, or believe that they're being persecuted. They may be very aggressive and even violent towards their babies. Some, on the other hand, neglect their babies entirely.

Obviously, these cases are very rare, and the vast majority of women who suffer in this way get the help they need. Most depressions of this sort are treated with *anti-depressant* drugs and these are said to work very well.

It goes without saying that a serious postnatal depression of this sort is enormously disruptive of family life. It puts a huge strain on the woman's partner and also her child, and women who've suffered in this way find that once they've recovered they've got a lot of catching up to do. They need a lot of help, sympathy and reassurance, and the sad fact is that some of them will be at a very high risk of falling prey to the illness if they have another baby. One in five mothers does have postnatal depression a second time; but at least that means four out of five get over it permanently.

Doctors have spent a lot of time trying to find out why postnatal depression happens, and have pointed the finger at many different things which seem to be related to it. First of all, some doctors have said that it's the result of a chemical imbalance in the brain triggered off by birth – could it be those hormones again? Some experts have pointed to the fact that women who have difficult pregnancies or births seem to be at a higher risk of becoming depressed, while others have said that being very young, having poor or inadequate housing and not having much money or security are the key factors.

It seems to me that one fact above all makes it likely that postnatal depression is probably the result of a combination of all these things and a few others – and that fact is that you're more likely to have postnatal depression if you're a first time mother, although it can happen to you after subsequent births.

Doctors who have made a study of depression divide it into two main categories, *endogenous* and *exogenous*. An endogenous depression is one which seems to come from within and have no cause; and exogenous depression is one which is a reaction to some outside event. Postnatal depression has been considered to be an *endogenous* depression, and it may well be so in some cases. But I believe that most postnatal depressions are the result of the simple fact that life changes dramatically when you have a baby.

Let me make this a little clearer. As we go through life, we come to events which represent major changes. It might be your first day at school, your first day at work, getting married, having a child, the death of a parent or retirement from work. These are transitions, life changing events. As they approach, and we know they're coming in most cases, we feel *anxious* about them; that is to say we feel worried and nervous about the effect of these events and what lies beyond them. Most of the things which happen in our lives are a mixture of good and bad, too; some of the experience is positive, some negative. We enjoy some of the things we gain, and regret some of the things we lose at every stage. This can be experienced as depression if, on balance, there is more of the negative than the positive about a particular transition in life.

It's my belief that the way society is organised guarantees that the experience of becoming a parent falls into that last category. Nearly everyone I've talked to would admit that during the early months and years of their children's lives they're more often depressed than not. Of course, it's a question of degree; some are, as we've seen, far more depressed than others. But I believe there is far more depression among young parents – and that the depressions last longer and are more serious than they should be. I think society could be changed in some fairly simple ways to make life easier and more satisfying for most young families.

Unhappy ever after?

It has been said that men never get postnatal depression, and that this proves the condition must be something to do with the hormones and chemicals in a woman's system. But men *do* get postnatal depression, even if their doctors persist in not calling it that.

Young fathers have their problems during both pregnancy and the early days of parenthood. They can be anxious and nervous, they can be tired, worried and feel burdened with responsibility. This is especially true of those young dads who suddenly find themselves the sole breadwinner in a family – that is, the partners of the young mums who decide to stay at home as full-time housewives and mothers.

I know that I was depressed when I went back to work and throughout the first year of Emma's life. I soon discovered that Sally felt very unhappy at home, and her depression made me feel very bad. The worst part of it all was that neither of us felt we could do anything about it. Sally neither wanted to go out to work nor believed that it was financially worthwhile, and I agreed with her. I had no way of staying at home more because there are just very few jobs around that would allow me to work from home, and I couldn't find one.

We also fell into the trap which claims many young couples, and with disastrous effect. I don't think we went out alone together more than once in the whole of Emma's first year, and our record in the years that followed hasn't been much better. We'd gone out quite a bit before Emma was born, but her birth was the effective end of our social life. That means we spent night after night indoors, watching the television, getting fed up, bored – and arguing – almost for want of something better to do. The fatigue and strain played their parts too, and when we look back we realise that what we really needed throughout that period was some time for each other and some time to ourselves.

It's a very easy trap to fall into. It's often difficult for young couples to find someone to look after the baby if they want to go out, especially when they're living a long way from family. That means making an effort to find someone reliable whom you can trust, and when you're already tired and under the stress of looking after a baby all day it's tempting simply not to bother. I have to say that most of the time you probably feel too tired to go out anyway, and you may well not be able to afford it either.

None the less, life can feel very dull and boring, and for many young fathers it can be worse than that. In a survey we ran in *Parents* magazine, it was discovered that a very large number of young fathers – perhaps even the majority – work extremely long hours. Some of them worked an average of 60, 70 or even 80 hours a week, and the reason was simple; they needed the money to support their families. Obviously, this means they're going to be very tired when they're at home.

So it's understandable that many young fathers might feel rather depressed after the birth of their children. You might therefore have a couple in which both partners are pretty miserable — and one more problem is going to add itself to their troubles. That's the great divide I was talking about earlier, the chasm between the worlds of work and home.

"John went off to work in the morning and came home late, tired out," said one young mother. "He was too tired to talk after his day's work, and I was too full of things to tell him to be able to get them out. It was worse when I'd had a bad day, too — then we were both like kids, ready to snap at each other at the slightest provocation."

The simple fact is that many couples find they're growing apart under the pressure of their separate worlds. It's a very common experience, and one Sally and I have gone through ourselves. If you've shared the pregnancy and birth, then you probably feel very close to each other at the beginning of parenthood. But you'll spend most of each day apart, and the time you're together will also be full of things which have to be done, all the paraphernalia and problems of living as a family, and running a household. Little by little the chasm between you grows, until one day you wake up and it seems that you're almost strangers.

This is a key source of the arguments which blight many a young couple's experience of parenthood, and also cause that dip in the amount of satisfaction with their marriages reported by many couples. Women complain that their partners don't listen to them, don't talk to them, aren't as attentive to them as they used to be. They also complain that they don't help with the housework or looking after the baby, and here the facts back them — in one survey I saw, it was said that one in four men have *never* changed their baby's nappies or looked after the baby alone for even an hour or so. Men also complain that their wives don't talk to them or understand their problems; they complain that their wives expect too much from them after a hard day's work, and both sexes complain that they don't get enough *appreciation* – from anybody.

It's very difficult to say with any accuracy whether these feelings have anything to do with marriages breaking up, but most people would say they do. I've said that having a baby puts an enormous strain on even the most stable of relationships, and obviously, if this divide between a couple is allowed to get wider, it's likely to end in separation and divorce. Many couples say that things started to go wrong in their marriages after the children came along; it's not the individual child's personal fault, she didn't ask to be brought into the world, after all. It's the pressure which does the damage.

Another problem with which all this is linked is violence in the family. There's been a lot of publicity in recent years about both wife and baby battering, and in many cases these terrible tragedies are the result of the sort of pressure I've been talking about. Most parents – when pressed – would admit that there have been times when they felt very violent towards their children, even tiny babies. There is violence in all of us, and it sometimes needs very little to bring it out. Imagine being woken every night – and kept awake for a long time – by the screaming of a baby, and you'll see how easy it is to feel this way. It's perfectly normal to feel hostile towards your children sometimes – although it's hard to admit.

Most parents, I'm relieved to say, resist the temptation to be violent towards their children. Some don't, and hurt their children, sometimes quite badly. The parents who do this were often treated violently themselves as children, and the real tragedy is that by doing it to the next generation, they're making it more likely that *their* children will be violent towards their offspring, and so on. Some men are also violent towards their wives, and again, there's often a history of violence, poverty and heavy drinking in their families.

Of course problems like these are much more complicated than I can explain here. But there does seem to be a connection in all this between your circumstances and the risks you run of being treated or acting in this way. This brings us back to the point that if you *choose* to become a parent at the right time, financially and emotionally as well as physically, and you consciously prepare yourself for parenthood and all it entails, you've got a much better chance of avoiding all these problems. The marriages which break up are often those which get off to a bad start, with a baby too soon and not enough money coming in. All those factors I talked about which are thought to be involved in postnatal depression are also linked to family violence. Of course, even the wealthiest and most secure couples sometimes get divorced, and it has to be said that the same sort of people are often involved in family violence. Having a baby puts an enormous amount of pressure on you, though — and if your circumstances make that pressure even greater, then you're taking a much bigger risk of ending up as a statistic in the divorce, depression or violence figures.

Money, money, money – again

One thing which often comes between couples is money. "The worst thing about giving up work was not having any money of my own any more," one woman said. "I'd lost all my independence, and I hated it. Pete said that the money he earned was ours, but I couldn't feel that way. It was his, he earned it, and now I had to ask him for money whenever I needed any — that made me feel very dependent."

This is a problem for most women who give up going out to work to look after their babies; apart from simply having less money coming into the house, they have none of their own, either. It can be very galling for a woman to be reduced to asking for the housekeeping money, and many men don't like being put into the position of looking after the family finances exclusively either. Again, it's something you can't really avoid if you choose this way of arranging your life.

There are other ways of doing that. One which is becoming very common is for the woman to go back to work quite soon after she has her baby. This means, of course, that she has to find someone to look after the baby while she's at work, and there are various ways of arranging this. Some women go back to work full-time and employ a live-in *nanny*, although this is very expensive; others put their children in a *nursery*, where they're looked after by a qualified children's nurse; others use a *childminder*, a woman who looks after one or more children in her own home. In Britain these have to be registered with the local authority, and they're subject to strict health and safety regulations.

Women working while their babies are very young aren't really a new development at all; poor women the world over have had to do it for centuries, simply because they needed the money. For most women that's still the main reason for going back to work today, and the number of women all over the world who are doing so is growing all the time. In fact, in recent years, the number of women who stay at home full-time to look after their children has fallen so far that they're now the minority.

What's different is that some women are actually choosing to go back to work after the birth for another reason, and that is simply to avoid the problems facing mothers at home. These women are the products of the feminist revolution, women who want to pursue careers and feel that there's more to life than just being a housewife and mother. They're the women who have broken out of the conditioning I described in Chapter 2, and who are continuing to help break it down.

That's not to say that they don't face enormous problems – they do, as do any women who go back to work and have their children cared for by someone else. The first problem for many families who take this way is a simple, practical one. If you want to go back to work, then there must be facilities for childcare available – and sometimes this just isn't the case. It means that very often children end up being looked after by unqualified childminders or relatives.

What's happened is that society hasn't kept pace with women's wants and needs. Many of the developed countries now have enshrined in their law the right for women to go back to work after they have a baby – but not all countries have provided enough childcare. In Britain, for example, if a woman has worked for the same employer for at least two years, she can leave work eleven weeks before her baby is due and stay off work until twenty nine weeks after the birth. Her job must be kept open for her, and she's paid a percentage of her wage for six weeks. In the vast majority of cases, it's illegal to dismiss a woman simply because she's become pregnant.

Britain is, in fact, a long way behind some other countries in terms of *maternity leave*. For example, women in France get a much better deal, with more money and more time off, and the same is true of several other countries. What we don't have in Britain – and again, this is found elsewhere – is a state system of childcare facilities. Families have to find their own solution to a very difficult problem, and it's a continual worry for many women who work – especially those without much money, which is most of them. That's the reason they have to go to work, after all.

Working mothers have other problems, too, not the least of which is guilt about what they're doing. Our society tends to think of women as childbearers and child raisers, not as people who work or who want to have careers. Women themselves are sometimes riddled with this sort of conditioning, and deep down believe that they should be at home looking after the children; the end result is guilt.

It's often seemed to me that women can't win whatever they do. I have used the word *appreciation* and it's a very important one in this context. My wife doesn't have a job, but if someone asks me whether she *works* or not, I don't say no – I say yes, because she works very hard keeping our household running and looking after the children while I go to work. I also used the phrase 'just a housewife and mother', and it's that word 'just' which says it all. Many people think that being a housewife and mother isn't important, valuable work; that because she's at home, my wife doesn't fill a demanding role with its own pressures and rewards. As you'll realise by now, that's completely the wrong way of looking at it, and it's the basic, root cause of all the problems I've been talking about in this chapter. As a parent, you're not *appreciated* – as a full-time occupation it's considered very lowly.

The freedom to choose

When you look at the law relating to maternity leave in Britain, you discover very quickly that one whole group of people is completely ignored in it – and that's fathers. There is, in fact, no provision for *paternity leave* in the United

Kingdom, and the same applies to many countries. By this, I mean an entitlement to some paid time off when a man becomes a father, which isn't counted as holiday or sick leave – that is, which doesn't mean he ends up with less time off in total, as I did after my children were born.

But in a recent report from the Equal Opportunities Commission, a body set up to make recommendations aimed at ensuring more equality for women with men, it was said that nine out of ten British fathers take time off work when their babies are born. Most of the men in the survey which formed the basis of the report also said that they thought a system of paternity leave was a necessity, and that they were very unhappy with society for forcing them back to work too soon. Our system of parental leave after a birth keeps the old ways going. It makes it almost impossible for fathers to take a large part in the early months of their children's lives, and therefore puts all the pressure on women. There's more, too. How many men in Britain today – or in other countries, for that matter – could get time off work because their children are ill? How many men could get the day off to visit their child's school to talk to the teacher? The answer is very few, and those who could would probably be made to feel a little guilty, to say the least.

That's because society is still overwhelmingly geared to the idea of men working and women staying at home. Men aren't expected to want to play a large part in their families, and to a great extent, women are still expected to subordinate their careers, jobs and outside interests to their families – women are still expected to come second. In a family where both partners work, it's more likely to be the mum who takes time off when a child is ill or on holiday from school and no one else can be found to look after her.

Of course, the blame for this state of affairs can't all be laid at society's door. Society is made up of individual people, and many men are reluctant to take a larger share in looking after the children. They are often reluctant to run the risk of slipping back in their careers which being more involved with the family might entail. This does happen, and you can see its effects on the career prospects of women. A woman who leaves work – for however long, whether it's a year, three years or ten years – often finds that she never catches up. The fact that she has missed those years will always mean that she's behind others who didn't – and that can even happen to women of great talent and drive.

Things are changing, though – but slowly. More women are pursuing careers outside the home, and it's interesting to see that more men are becoming more involved in their families. It seems as if the people on both sides of the great divide between work and home are trying to build bridges across it to each other. I'm one of the many men who would like to spend more time with my family, and there are many women who would like to have a better career with wider opportunities. What many of us are looking for is a way of life in which we could combine, in which we could share both the benefits of having children and the burdens, and also in which we could share the pleasures and problems of work.

One other element in all this is the growing level of unemployment in many countries brought about by economic recession and technological change. In the age of computers and dole queues, many families find that life is suddenly topsy turvy anyway, with fathers at home and mothers going out to work. This sort of pressure is leading to change in our attitudes, although we've still got a long way to go.

You should keep one point in mind in this connection – and it's that if you want to keep your options open, it's worth thinking about work and your future at a time when you can still do something about it. What I mean is that even if you know you want to have children and stay at home to look after them full-time while they're small, it's still a good idea to think about a career which you could return to in later years. Even if you have a baby at twenty and stay at home for twenty years, there's still a large part of your life left to fill after that. Many older women do find life very difficult after their children leave home, especially if they have nothing else to devote themselves to.

And even if you know your career is going to be important to you and that you're going to work when your children are young, it's still sensible to take steps to make sure you can minimise the disruption and problems. That might mean getting extra qualifications and staying on longer at school, or even going to college. It might mean waiting a little longer to start having a family, maybe even until you're in your thirties – something a growing number of women are doing. It means you can leave work at a time when you're more established – and can therefore return more easily.

Some people become single parents by choice; a girl might not want to marry the father of her baby or even live with him. Others have little choice about it, if their marriages split up and they're left holding the baby. But however a person becomes a single parent, life will be hard. If they don't work, they'll have to live on welfare benefits, and that means they'll have very little money. If they want to work, they'll have to find a job and childcare – and then keep everything going with very little support. It's hard enough for working parents who've got a partner, but for a single parent a child with a cough or cold can represent near disaster.

I'm full of admiration for single parents, and that's because they're often very courageous as well as being at the forefront of some of the developments which will help all parents in the long run. Groups of single parents have agitated and forced local councils to provide more childcare facilities. They've forced employers to be more flexible in their attitudes, and they're pioneering new ideas like *jobsharing*. In this, two parents share one job, perhaps doing half a day each, or half a week each, and share the care of the children too. It doesn't cost the employer any more – and he still gets the job done. It's the sort of thing I think we're going to see more of in the future, especially if unemployment remains as high as it is now.

Other parents are joining in, too, in the search for a better deal. There are couples now where mothers and fathers have swapped roles, with the father staying at home to look after the children and the mother going out to work. Interestingly enough, many of these fathers (although their total number isn't large) suffer the same sort of problems that mothers at home do; they feel under-valued, bored, depressed and so on. They also have the problem that many people think they're mad or just plain lazy. After all, they say, being a 'housewife' isn't a *manly* thing to do.

What all these developments mean is that people are trying to break down old ways of doing things. In Chapter 2 I talked about the freedom to *choose* parenthood, and what these people are doing is working for more freedom. The problems of becoming a parent are made easier to bear if it's an experience which is shared, and I believe society could change in a few simple ways to make that sharing easier. Introducing real paternity leave in Britain would make families happier and ease the problems of the early months, so long as it was long enough. Giving parents more flexibility so that they could both take time off for family problems or for things like visits to schools would promote more equality between mothers and fathers. Measures like these would make for happier parents – and happier children.

These things have already been introduced in countries more progressive than Britain. For example, in Sweden, each parent is entitled to up to six months' leave after the birth of a child. This can be taken by both parents together, or it can be split up, or taken one lot after the other. Parents in West Germany – either the mother or father – are entitled to up to five days paid leave a year to care for a sick child. Other benefits are also higher in other countries, and France has taken the enlightened step of making a very high maternity grant payable on the condition that you go to all your antenatal check-ups. A simple measure that promotes good health in a very direct way.

You and your future

Of course one major problem is that for those of you who are on the verge of taking this giant step into parenthood, much of what I've written about in this section isn't going to be much better for many years to come. The sort of attitudes I've been talking about are very deeply engrained and slow to change. Even in progressive Sweden, many men don't take their full allocation of paternity leave and their wives take the burden of childcare. That's because although it's available to them, they've still grown up in a society which at its roots is still very traditional.

But at least Swedish men have got the opportunity, and it's likely that more men will do something about it in the years to come. Changes of this kind have to start in the cradle, almost. As fathers take more part in bringing up their children, so their sons will grow up more used to the idea of men as parents, and it's likely that sharing family life will be more natural to them. The same is true of daughters who grow up in households where their mothers have broader interests and perhaps a career. I hope that one day we *all* will be able to share *all* the good things in life – and help each other with the bad.

And what about you? How will it all affect you? I'll just emphasise one thing, and it's very simple. Most people do survive parenthood, and even go on – like us – to have more children, although having read this far you'll probably think they're crazy. But having a second child is usually easier all round; you're used to all the sorts of problems I've talked about, you're probably on the way to working out what you want in life, and things are a bit clearer. You'll also probably have a little more stamina – and be less inclined to worry so much. I can do no better than quote a reader who was interviewed in *Parents* and who said very simply: "With your first baby you break your heart. With your second you break the rules."

The choice is yours, as I said right at the beginning, and I hope that by now you understand that how you handle that decision is very important. It's also important that you should carve out the way of life *you* want, and that means being sure you know what you want from the start. And if you're one of the people who does that, you'll be helping to make sure the changes I've talked about come a little sooner.

Last Words

10. Is it worth it?

IT'S TAKEN me five months to write this book, and all the time I've been slaving over my steaming typewriter I've been wondering how on earth I would bring it to an end. I want very much to leave you on a positive note.

You've heard all about the difficulties involved in becoming a parent. You know now that if you take this step there will be times when you'll be frustrated, exhausted, depressed, anxious, worried, bored and many other things. I've painted as complete – and as realistic – a picture as I can, and I've set out deliberately to shatter any illusions about parenthood you might have.

So why should you bother to have children at all? How can I say anything now which will convince you that it's worth doing?

The first thing to say is that I don't want to persuade anybody to do anything they're not suited to. Now you know about parenthood, it's up to you to make the decision. If you choose not to have children, then that's fine – and no one on this planet should be allowed to make you feel guilty or inadequate in any way for doing so. In some ways you're taking one of the most difficult paths of all – the path which has no direction but the one you choose. People with children have much of their future path mapped out for them.

If you decide that you want to have children, then let me stress for one last time the importance of making that decision for the right reasons and taking positive steps to ensure you give yourself the best chance of doing it right. Look after your health, try to make sure that you're starting from a sound economic base, and don't be afraid to seek help at any stage for any problem. There is no need to suffer alone, and in some cases that's the worst thing you could possibly do. Finally, be prepared to feel very negative about it all. Be ready to go through hell, and always remember that even those people who seem to have done all the right preparation and have everything going for them sometimes crack under the strain. That doesn't mean their lives have to be ruined – but becoming a parent is a process which involves an enormous amount of pressure, and no one knows how they're going to cope with it until the day comes when they have to.

But one thing I do know; most of you will become parents anyway, whatever I've said. I hope that reading this book will help you to enjoy the experience and also to avoid some of the problems Sally and I and many other couples have had to face. But the instinctive, biological urge to reproduce yourself is very powerful. It's something which overwhelms many of us in the end, and the important thing is to make sure that we retain some control at least over the circumstances in which it does.

I thought of leaving you with a long list of all the good things about having children. That would mean talking about all sorts of intangible things, like the wonder you feel when you hold your child in your arms for the very first time; the awe you feel at the process of birth; the pride you feel as your child reaches and passes through a different stage, stages like learning to walk or going to school. It's very difficult to do that without tumbling over a precipice and into the depths of sentimentality; it's also difficult to avoid drifting into some of the rosy illusions I've been trying to shatter. Amidst the chaos and the dirty nappies, the problems over money and work, we parents still have a tendency to go gooey-eyed over babies and soft-hearted over our children. That's part of what's good about the experience.

Something else intangible is the sense of growth and change parenthood brings, something which has been very important to me. In a very simple sense, my life has grown with my children; every day is different, every minute brings new challenges and triumphs. A smile from Thomas, my youngest child; a new picture from Emma, one which shows that she has a real talent for drawing; a long conversation with Helen which reveals her to be articulate, warm and friendly, even at three years old.

Is it all worth it? Is parenthood worth the sleepless nights and the worry? For it has to be said that Sally and I worry about our children all the time and that essentially we're hostages to their good health and future. We are anxious about every minute of their lives, and spend much time wondering what that future will bring them.

And I have to say, yes – it *is* worth it. I love my children, and the strange thing now is that I can't imagine what life without them would be like. My children make the world a better, a happier place for me. They make me see things more clearly, they make me enjoy life more at the same time as they keep me short of money and awake at night.

What more can I say than that each of our children has brought more love into the world for us? And if this book helps you to make sure that your experience of being a parent increases the amount of love in *your* life, then I'll be more than happy. I wish you all the luck and love in the world – you're going to need them both!

THERE ARE various organisations in Britain which might be able to help you at different stages of the process of becoming a parent.

Foresight is the short name of The Association for the Promotion of Pre-conceptual Care. It's based at Woodhurst, Hydestile, Godalming, Surrey GU9 4OY.

The National Childbirth Trust at 9 Queensborough Terrace, London W2 3TB, is a national charity which offers help to couples who are having a baby.

The Maternity Alliance at 309 Kentish Town Road, London NW5, is a campaigning group for maternity rights and welfare.

Useful books

Pregnancy by Gordon Bourne (Pan); still one of the most comprehensive books around.

The Childbirth Book by Christine Beels (Granada); very good on labour and birth; feminist and pro-natural birth in about equal measure.

The Experience of Childbirth by Sheila Kitzinger (Penguin); Sheila Kitzinger, one of the leading writers about birth today, has written many books about it and related matters such as *The Experience of Breastfeeding* (Penguin) and *The New Good Birth Guide* (Penguin).

Breast is Best by Drs Penny and Andrew Stanway (Pan); this is the definitive book about breastfeeding, matched only by *The Breastfeeding Book* by Màire Messenger Davies (Century) in recent years.

Babyhood and *Baby and Child* by Penelope Leach (both Penguin).

How to Survive as a Working Mother by Lesley Garner (Penguin).

Index

Note: page numbers in italics refer to illustrations.

Abdomen 66, 68, 70, 77
Abortion 28, 29–30, 76, 77–8
Abscess, breast 128
Adoption 29, 30
Afterbirth 91, 105, *see also* Placenta
Age, and pregnancy 28, 45–6
Alcohol, alcoholism 32, 40–1
Allergies 36, 125–6
Amniotic fluid, sac 60, 64, 80, 92, 98; amniocentesis 77–8
Anaemia 35, 36, 77
Anaesthetics 99, 102, 107
Anorexia nervosa 37
Antenatal care 76–82, 87, 106, 109, *see also* Preconceptual care
Antenatal classes 79, 80, 85, 94
Anxiety 170; and breastfeeding 110, 127; in expectant fathers 83, 84, 170; in pregnancy 73, 74, 79, 94
Apgar score 105
Appearance: baby's 111; in pregnancy 72–3, 81; society's attitudes towards 37, 125
Areolae 69, 127

Baby battering 173
Baby blues, *see* Depression, post-natal

Back strain, in pregnancy 70
Bath, baby's 119–20
Behaviour, children's 126, 153–5, 157
Birth canal 91
Bladder: baby's control of 118, 156; in pregnancy 68
Blood levels, in pregnancy 69, 80, *see also* Anaemia
Blood pressure 36, 77, 87–8
Blood tests, in pregnancy 77
Bonding 99, 104, 106, 107, 128
Books, children's 147
Boredom, mother's 167
Bottle feeding 110, 124–5, 126, 129–30
Bowel movements 34, 38, 70, 98; baby's control of 111, 118–9, 156
Boys: and puberty 52; social conditioning of 21, 83, 147–8
Brain: damage 159, 160; development of 65–6, 147
Braxton-Hicks contractions 92
Breast feeding 82, 99, 105, 107, 124–30 *passim*; and love life 132; and postnatal depression 109–10
Breathing: and childbirth 79, 94, 102; foetal 64; new baby's 90, 99, 104, 105; in pregnancy 69, 70
Breech presentation 106–7
Brow presentation 106

Caesarean births 95, 100, 106, 107
Calcium, dietary 36
Carbohydrates, dietary 35
Care: antenatal 76–82, 87, 106, 109; child 44–5, 147, 174–6, 177, 179; of new baby 79, 118–30, 134–5; post-natal 130–2, 136; preconceptual 32–47 *passim*
Cervix 55, 59, 88–9, 91, 92
Childbirth 18–9, 38, 74, 90–113; and postnatal depression 169; preparation for 79, 85, 94
Childminders 134, 175
Chromosomes 52–4, 58
Clinics: antenatal 76–8, 109; well baby 159
Colostrum 81, 110
Conception, *see* Fertilisation
Constipation 34, 70, 82
Contraception 17–8, 28, 31, 128
Contractions 91, 92–3, 110
Cost of having a baby 22–4
Cramp, in pregnancy 70, 80
Crawling 144–5
Crying, baby's 104, 118, 128

Deafness, in children 159
Death, and childbirth 18–9, 87, 101
Delivery 91, 98–9, 100, 103–4; of afterbirth 91, 105; breech 106–7; by

Caesarean 95, 100, 106, 107
Depression 29, 82, 89, 108, 170–2; postnatal 26, 100, 109, 110–11, 168–70, 174
Development: child 18, 66, 139–61, 163; embryonic, foetal 40–1, 58–67, 77, 141
Diet 32, 33–6; and breastfeeding 130; children's 157; and pregnancy 33, 35, 37, 70, 81; and stretch marks 71–2
Dilation, of cervix 91, 92
Discipline 155
Discomfort, in pregnancy 70–1, 80
Divorce 30, 45, 173, 174
Doctors, and antenatal care 76, 78–9; and childbirth 96–7, 101, 102
Dreams 66–7, 74
Drugs 41, 62, 95, 99, 101–2, 108

Eczema 126
Egg, see Ovum
Ejaculation 54, 55
Embryo 58–61
Emotions 103–4, 109, 110–12, 140; father's 82–5, 96, 104; and parenthood 123–4; and pregnancy 72–5, 85–7
Endometrium 55, 56
Enjoyment, of pregnancy 75, 85–7
Entonox 99
Epididymis 52
Epidural anaesthetics 99, 102, 107
Episiotomy 98, 101, 106, 131
Exercise 32, 38–9, 43–4; antenatal 38, 71, 81; postnatal 131–2

Fallopian tubes 51, 52, 54, 55, 57, 59
Family, the 18, 19, 24–5, 139–40

Family planning, see Contraception
Fashion, and pregnancy 73
Fat, dietary 33–4, 36
Fathers, as breadwinner 18, 20, 22, 85, 162, 163–4, 171–2; and child care 44, 134–5, 147, 177, 178; depression in 82, 170–2; jealousy of new baby 84, 133; paternity leave 133, 176–7, 180; presence at birth 95–6, 104; reaction to pregnancy 30, 82–5; relationship with mother 44–6, 82–5, 132–5; society's expectations of 20, 22
Fear, in pregnancy 74, 79, 94
Feeding, see Bottle feeding; Breast feeding; Solid feeds
Fertilisation 17, 51–6 passim, 58; fertility problems 56–8
Fibre, dietary 34, 70
Foetus 39–42, 60, 61–7, 141
Folic acid 35, 77
Forceps 99
Foresight (The Association for the Promotion of Preconceptual Care) 188

Gas and oxygen 99
Genes 52–3, 58; genetic counselling 46–7
Genitals, see Sex organs
German measles 42, 62, 77, 108
Girls, puberty in 52, 56; social conditioning of 21, 83, 147–8, 163
Going out, parents need to 171; with baby 165–6
Grief, and miscarriage, stillbirth 89, 108
Guilt 74, 111, 112, 176; and abortion, adoption 29, 30; and

bottle feeding 110 129

Haemophilia 46
Haemorrhoids 34, 70
Hair care, in pregnancy 81
Hand-eye coordination 143–4, 149
Hand play 148
Handicapped baby 1 causes 41, 42, 62, 160; detection 77–109; parental fear of 74
Head, baby's: birth of 91; engagement of 106; support of 119
Head control, development of 143, 144
Health 32–47, 159–6
Health visitors 136,
Hearing, baby's 141, 142, 159; in womb 64
Heart beat: foetal 77 pregnancy 64–5, 6
Heart disorders 32, 3 34, 35, 36, 38
Heartburn, in pregnancy 70
Hereditary disorders 46–7
Home confinement 102–3
Hormones: and breast feeding 128; and infertility 57; and labour 91; and postnatal depressior 110, 169; in pregnancy 68, 69, 70, 7 75; and stress 65
Hospital confinement 97–100, 101–2, 109–
Hyperactivity, in children 126

Illness: in children 4 160–1, and diet 32– passim; hereditary 46–7; and smoking 32–3, 39–40
Immunisations 42, 1
Induction, of labour 97–8, 101

Index

Infertility 37, 56–8
Inheritance 24, 32, 52–3, 140; and illness 46–7; and stretch marks 71
Insomnia 43, 80, 82
Intellectual development 66, 140, 141, 147
Iron, dietary 36, 77
Isolation: and fathers 84, 112; and mothers 164–5, 168

Jealousy 84, 133

Labour 90–103 passim, 106–7; preparation for 79, 85, 94
Language development 141, 142, 145–7, 159
Let-down reflex 128
Linea negra 69
Lochia 131
Love, need for 25, 45, 159

Marriage 30; stress in 45, 84–5, 172–3, 174
Mastitis 128
Maternity Alliance 188
Maternity leave 175–6, 180
Measurements, of new baby 105
Meconium 111, 118
Men, see also Fathers; society's attitudes towards 20, 22, 177
Menarche 56
Menopause 56
Menstruation 37, 56, 57, 59, see also Ovulation; and breastfeeding 128; after childbirth 131
Midwives, and antenatal care 76, 78, 79; and childbirth 96–7, 101, 102
Minerals 36, see also Zinc
Miscarriage 88–9, 108
Morning sickness 69
Moro reflex, see Startle reflex
Mothers, care of after childbirth 130–2; and child development 163; death from childbirth 18–9, 87; feelings of 72, 74, 85–7, 103–4, 109, see also Anxiety, Depression etc; housebound 20, 162, 163, 164–7, 168; isolation of 164–5, 168; loss of independence 174; maternity leave 175–6, 180; physical stress of 18; relationship with child 99, 104, 106, 107, 128, 130, 135; relationship with father 44–6, 82–5, 132–5; society's expectations of 20, 21, 125; unmarried 28–9, 179; and unwanted pregnancies 29, 30; working 21–2, 134, 162, 163, 174–6, 177–9

Movement, development of 141, see also Crawling; Hand-eye coordination; Walking; foetal 63
Mucus plug 55, 92

Nannies 174
National Childbirth Trust 79, 188
Nausea, and pregnancy 69, 70, 74, 75, 80, 82
Nightmares, in pregnancy 74
Nipples 81–2, 127
Nurseries 134, 174

Oestrogen 52, 55, 68
Ovaries 51, 52, 59
Ovulation 52–8 passim, 68, 128
Ovum, ova 17, 51–60 passim, see also Ovulation

Pain, and childbirth 93–6, 99, 101–2
Parents, parenthood 137–8, 185–7, see also Fathers; Mothers; and child development 139–40, 145–8, 152–61 passim; choices, reasons for having baby 17–31; financial pressures 22–4, 30, 174; health 32–47 passim; and new baby 117–24, 135–6, 142–3; relationship between 44–6, 82–5, 132–5; single 28, 29, 179; stresses, strains of 18–9, 45, 85, 133, 171–4, 185–6; traditional attitudes towards 19–21, 162–3, 177, 178, 180; and violence 30, 173, 174
Paternity leave 133, 176–7, 180
Pelvic floor 131
Penis 51, 55
Periods, see Menstruation
Personality, development of 66, 140
Pethidine 99
Piles 34, 70
Pill, the, see Contraceptive pill
Pituitary gland 52, 91
Placenta 60, 64, 80, 90, 91, 105
Play 148–53, see also Toys
Positions, of baby in womb 106–7; for childbirth 98–9
Postnatal care 130–2, 136
Preconceptual care 32–47 passim
Pre-eclampsia 88
Pregnancy 28, 32–47 passim, 68–89, 169; development of baby in 59–67; termination of 29–30
Premature babies 107–8
Preparation, for childbirth and parenthood 21, 83, 94, 101–2
Progesterone 55, 68, 71
Protein 35
Puberty 52, see also Menarche
Pubococygeus muscles 131–2

Index

Punishment, and children 155

Quickening 63

Rashes, and pregnancy 70, 81
Reflexes: baby's 105, 119, 141, 142; and breastfeeding 128
Rejection, of baby 95, 168–9
Relaxation 43–4; and childbirth 79
Role-playing 148, 149, 151
Rooting reflex 141
Roughage, dietary 34, 70
Rubella, see German measles

Salt, and blood pressure 36
Security, child's need for 45
Semen 55
Seminal vesicles 52, 55
Seminiferous tubules 52
Sex chromosomes 52, 53–4
Sex organs 51, 57, 59, 61
Sexual intercourse 17, 18, 26, 54–5, 57; after childbirth 132–3; in pregnancy 86–7
Shirodkar stitch 89
'Shotgun' weddings 30
Shopping, with baby 165, 166
Show, and onset of labour 91–2
Sickness, see Nausea
Single parent families 28, 29, 179
Sitting up 144
Skin, and excema 126; of new baby 105; and pregnancy 69, 70, 71–2, 81
Sleep 38, 44, see also Insomnia; and new baby 118, 157–8
Slimming 37
Smacking 155
Smell, baby's sense of 141

Smoking 32; in pregnancy 33, 39–40
Social life, parents need for 171
Social play 148, 150, 151
Solid feeds 129, 156
Speech development, see Language development
Sperms 51–5 passim, 57, 58
Squatting, and childbirth 99
Standing up 144
Startle reflex 119, 142
Stillbirth 19, 108
Stress 32, 42–4, 45; foetal 65; and parenthood 85, 133, 172–3, 174; and pregnancy 82–4
Stretch marks 71–2, 80
Sucking, baby's 64, 105, 129, 141; and milk supply 110, 127
Sugar, in diet 34
Swelling, of hands, feet 88

Talking, see also Language development; to baby 106, 142
Tantrums 154
Taste, and new baby 141
Teenagers, and pregnancy 28
Teeth, development of 156–7
Test tube baby technique 57
Testicles 51, 52, 57
Tests, for and during pregnancy 75, 77, 88
Thalidomide 41, 108
Thrush, in pregnancy 70
Tiredness, and pregnancy 69, 70, 74, 75, 80, 82
Toilet training 156
Toys 21, 83, 150–2
Twin pregnancies 53

Ultrasound 77
Umbilical cord 60, 64, 90, 91, 104; stump 105, 111, 119
Unemployment, and family life 178

Unmarried mothers 28, 29, 179
Urination, in pregnancy 68
Urine tests 75, 77, 88
Uterus, see Womb

Vacuum extractors 100
Vagina 51, 54, 55, 59, 131, 132
Varicose veins 34, 70, 71
Vas deferens 52
Vernix 104
Violence, family 30, 173, 174
Vision, baby's 141, 142, 143–4, 149
Vitamins 35–6, 44
Vomiting, and pregnancy 69, 82

Walking, development of 140, 141, 144–5; reflex in new baby 142
Waters, bag of, see Amniotic fluid
Weaning 156
Weight: baby's 80; child's 157; and diet 33; and exercise 38; gain in pregnancy 68, 71, 77, 80–1; loss after childbirth 130–1, 135; loss by slimming 37
Well baby clinics 159
Whooping cough immunisation 160
Wind, in pregnancy 70
Womb 51, 55, 56, see also Cervix; baby's 111; after childbirth 110; and labour 91–3, 97; position of baby in 106–7; and pregnancy 59–67, 68, 80
Women, see also Mothers; society's attitudes towards 20, 21–2, 125, 163, 166, 175–6, 177

X-rays, and pregnancy 62, 76

Zinc, and stretch marks 71–2